Teen Health Series

# Abuse And Violence Information For Teens, Second Edition

# Abuse And Violence Information For Teens, Second Edition

Health Tips About The Causes
And Consequences Of Abusive
And Violent Behavior

Including Facts About The Types Of Abuse
And Violence, The Warning Signs Of Abusive
And Violent Behavior, Health Concerns Of Victims,
And Getting Help And Staying Safe

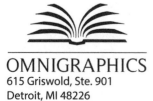

OMNIGRAPHICS
615 Griswold, Ste. 901
Detroit, MI 48226

Bibliographic Note
Because this page cannot legibly accommodate all the copyright notices, the Bibliographic Note portion of the
Preface constitutes an extension of the copyright notice.

\* \* \*

Omnigraphics
a part of Relevant Information
Keith Jones, *Managing Editor*

\* \* \*

Library of Congress Cataloging-in-Publication Data

Names: Omnigraphics, Inc., issuing body.

Title: Abuse and violence information for teens: health tips about the causes and consequences
of abusive and violent behavior including facts about the types of abuse and violence, the
warning signs of abusive and violent behavior, health concerns of victims, and getting help and
staying safe.

Description: Detroit, MI: Omnigraphics, [2017] | Series: Teen health series | Includes
bibliographical references and index.

Identifiers: LCCN 2016049906 (print) | LCCN 2016055647 (ebook) | ISBN 9780780814561
(hardcover: alk. paper) | ISBN 9780780814554 (ebook) | ISBN 9780780814554 (eBook)

Subjects: LCSH: Youth and violence--United States--Juvenile literature. | Youth and
violence--United States--Prevention--Juvenile literature.

Classification: LCC HQ799.2.V56 A25 2017 (print) | LCC HQ799.2.V56 (ebook) | DDC 303.60835--
dc23

LC record available at https://lccn.loc.gov/2016049906

# Table of Contents

# Part Three: Recognizing And Treating The Consequences Of Abuse And Violence

# Part Four: Prevention, Staying Safe, And Your Legal Rights As A Victim

# Part Five: If You Need More Information

# Preface

## About This Book

Teens experience violence in many forms, including bullying, fighting, hazing, dating violence, sexual abuse, domestic violence, and even homicide. According to a 2015 report from Centers for Disease Control and Prevention (CDC), 4,787 young people aged 10 to 24 years were victims of homicide—an average of 13 each day. Although media coverage often focuses on shootings, other types of violence impact greater numbers of teens. In fact, according to the same report over 599,000 young people aged 10 to 24 years had physical assault injuries treated in U.S. emergency departments—an average of 1,642 each day. The physical and emotional scars resulting from these experiences can endure for a lifetime.

*Abuse And Violence Information For Teens*, Second Edition, discusses contributing factors and warning signs for the most commonly experienced types of abuse and violence. Facts about seeking medical care and mental health services for the physical and emotional consequences are also included. A section on prevention and safety suggests ways teens can help prevent violence and offers guidelines for staying out of harm's way. In addition, information about victims' rights is provided, and the book concludes with a resource section featuring statistical data, directories of organizations and agencies able to offer assistance, and suggestions for additional reading.

## How To Use This Book

This book is divided into parts and chapters. Parts focus on broad areas of interest; chapters are devoted to single topics within a part.

*Part One: Types Of Abuse* provides information on domestic violence, child abuse, elder abuse, sibling abuse, sexual abuse, incest, stalking, and sexual harassment. It also discusses the role new technologies play in child pornography and sexual exploitation.

*Part Two: Violence And The Teen Experience* begins with a discussion regarding possible risk factors and warning signs for youth violence, including conduct disorders, electronic aggression, and substance abuse. It continues with facts about forms of violence teens often encounter. These include dating violence, bullying, hazing, and gang-related activity. The part concludes with facts about self-injury, suicide, and violence against the LGBT community.

*Part Three: Recognizing And Treating The Consequences Of Abuse And Violence* explains the aftermath and repercussions of traumatic experiences. It explains what to do after a sexual assault and discusses the potential long-term effects of child abuse and neglect. It also provides facts about depression, posttraumatic stress disorder, and other mental health issues related to the experience of abuse and violence.

*Part Four: Prevention, Staying Safe, And Your Legal Rights As A Victim* discusses what can be done to prevent abuse and violence and gives helpful information about how to stay safe in an abusive or violent situation. It concludes with facts about a victim's legal rights.

*Part Five: If You Need More Information* includes a statistical summary of abuse and violence, resource directories, and information on how and where to report child abuse.

# Bibliographic Note

This volume contains documents and excerpts from publications issued by the following U.S. government agencies: Administration for Children and Families (ACF); Centers for Disease Control and Prevention (CDC); Child Welfare Information Gateway; *Eunice Kennedy Shriver* National Institute of Child Health and Human Development (NICHD); Federal Bureau of Investigation (FBI); Library of Congress (LOC); National Criminal Justice Reference Service (NCJRS); National Institute of Justice (NIJ); National Institute of Mental Health (NIMH); National Institute on Drug Abuse (NIDA); National Oceanic and Atmospheric Administration (NOAA); National Sex Offender Public Website (NSOPW); Office of Juvenile Justice and Delinquency Prevention (OJJDP); Office on Women's Health (OWH); U.S. Department of Education (ED); U.S. Department of Health and Human Services (HHS); U.S. Department of Justice (DOJ); U.S. Department of Veterans Affairs (VA); U.S. Equal Employment Opportunity Commission (EEOC); U.S. House of Representatives; and Youth.gov.

In addition, this volume contains copyrighted documents from the following organization: The Nemours Foundation

It may also contain original material produced by Omnigraphics and reviewed by medical consultants.

The photograph on the front cover is © Antonio Guillem/iStock.

# Medical Review

Omnigraphics contracts with a team of qualified, senior medical professionals who serve as medical consultants for the *Teen Health Series*. As necessary, medical consultants review reprinted and originally written material for currency and accuracy. Citations including the phrase, Reviewed (month, year)" indicate material reviewed by this team. Medical consultation services are provided to the *Teen Health Series* editors by:

Dr. Senthil Selvan, MBBS, DCH, MD
Dr. K. Sivanandham, MBBS, DCH, MS (Research), PhD

## About The *Teen Health Series*

At the request of librarians serving today's young adults, the *Teen Health Series* was developed as a specially focused set of volumes within Omnigraphics' *Health Reference Series*. Each volume deals comprehensively with a topic selected according to the needs and interests of people in middle school and high school. Teens seeking preventive guidance, information about disease warning signs, medical statistics, and risk factors for health problems will find answers to their questions in the *Teen Health Series*. The *Series*, however, is not intended to serve as a tool for diagnosing illness, in prescribing treatments, or as a substitute for the physician/patient relationship. All people concerned about medical symptoms or the possibility of disease are encouraged to seek professional care from an appropriate healthcare provider.

If there is a topic you would like to see addressed in a future volume of the *Teen Health Series*, please write to:

Editor
*Teen Health Series*
Omnigraphics
615 Griswold, Ste. 901
Detroit, MI 48226

## A Note About Spelling And Style

*Teen Health Series* editors use *Stedman's Medical Dictionary* as an authority for questions related to the spelling of medical terms and the *Chicago Manual of Style* for questions related to grammatical structures, punctuation, and other editorial concerns. Consistent adherence is not always possible, however, because the individual volumes within the *Series* include many documents from a wide variety of different producers and copyright holders, and the editor's primary goal is to present material from each source as accurately as is possible following the terms specified by each document's producer. This sometimes means that information in different chapters or sections may follow other guidelines and alternate spelling authorities.

# Part One
Types Of Abuse

# Chapter 1
# Abuse In Families: An Overview

## What Is Abuse?

Abuse can be physical, sexual, emotional, verbal, or a combination of any or all of these. Abuse can also be neglect, which is when parents or guardians don't take care of the basic needs of the children who depend on them.

**Physical abuse** is often the most easily recognized form of abuse. Physical abuse can be any kind of hitting, shaking, burning, pinching, biting, choking, throwing, beating, and other actions that cause physical injury, leave marks, or cause pain.

**Sexual abuse** is any type of sexual contact between an adult and anyone younger than 18; between a significantly older child and a younger child; or if one person overpowers another, regardless of age. If a family member sexually abuses another family member, this is called incest.

**Emotional abuse** can be the most difficult to identify because there are usually no outward signs of the abuse. Emotional abuse happens when yelling and anger go too far or when parents constantly criticize, threaten, or dismiss kids or teens until their self-esteem and feelings of self-worth are damaged. Emotional abuse can hurt and cause damage just as physical abuse does.

**Neglect** is difficult to identify and define. Neglect occurs when a child or teen doesn't have adequate food, housing, clothes, medical care, or supervision. Emotional neglect happens when a parent doesn't provide enough emotional support or deliberately and consistently pays very little or no attention to a child. This doesn't mean that a parent doesn't give a kid

About This Chapter: Text in this chapter is excerpted from "Abuse," © 1995–2016. The Nemours Foundation/ KidsHealth®. Reprinted with permission.

something he or she wants, like a new computer or a cell phone, but refers to more basic needs like food, shelter, and love.

Family violence can affect anyone. It can happen in any kind of family. Sometimes parents abuse each other, which can be hard for a child to witness. Some parents abuse their kids by using physical or verbal cruelty as a way of discipline.

Abuse doesn't just happen in families, of course. Bullying is a form of abusive behavior. Bullying someone through intimidation, threats, or humiliation can be just as abusive as beating someone up. People who bully others may have been abused themselves. This is also true of people who abuse someone they're dating. But being abused is no excuse for abusing someone else.

Abuse can also take the form of hate crimes directed at people just because of their race, religion, abilities, gender, or sexual orientation.

# Recognizing Abuse

It may sound strange, but people sometimes have trouble recognizing that they are being abused. Recognizing abuse may be especially difficult for someone who has lived with it for many years. A person might think that it's just the way things are and that there's nothing that can be done. People who are abused might mistakenly think that it's their fault for not doing what their parents tell them, breaking rules, or not living up to someone's expectations.

Growing up in a family where there is violence or abuse can make a person think that is the right way or the only way for family members to treat each other. Somebody who has only known an abusive relationship might mistakenly think that hitting, beating, pushing, shoving, or angry name-calling are perfectly normal ways to treat someone when you're mad.

Seeing parents treat each other in abusive ways might lead a child to think that's OK in relationships. But abuse is not a typical or healthy way to treat people.

If you're not sure you are being abused, or if you suspect a friend is, it's always OK to ask a trusted adult or friend.

# Why Does Abuse Happen?

If you're one of the thousands of people living in an abusive situation, it can help to understand why some people abuse—and to realize that the abuse is *not your fault*. Sometimes abusers manipulate those they're abusing by telling them they did something wrong or "asked for it" in some way. But that's not true.

There is no single reason why people abuse others. But some factors seem to make it more likely that someone may lose control, yell, hit, or hurt.

Sometimes, growing up in an abusive family can lead a person to think that example is a good way to discipline others. Others become abusive because they're not able to manage their feelings properly. For example, someone who is unable to control anger or can't cope with stressful personal situations (like the loss of a job or marriage problems) may lash out at others inappropriately. Also, drinking too much and/or drug use can make it difficult for some people to control their actions.

Certain types of personality disorders or mental illness might also interfere with someone's ability to relate to others in healthy ways or cause problems with aggression or self-control. Of course, not everyone with a personality disorder or mental illness becomes abusive.

Fortunately, people who abuse can get help and learn how to take responsibility for how they act—and learn ways to stop.

## What Are The Effects Of Abuse?

When people are abused, it can affect every aspect of their lives, especially self-esteem. How much harm is done often depends on the situation and sometimes on how severe the abuse is. Sometimes a seemingly minor thing can trigger a big reaction. Being touched inappropriately by a family member, or being told to keep secrets, for example, can be very confusing and traumatic.

Every family has arguments. Friends, couples, coaches, and teachers can get upset, frustrated, or have a bad day. We all go through difficult times when someone is stressed and angry. Punishments and discipline—like removing privileges, grounding, or being sent to your room—are common.

Yelling and anger can happen in lots of parent–teen relationships and in friendships—although it can feel pretty bad to have an argument with a parent or friend. But if punishments, arguments, or yelling go too far or last too long it can lead to stress and other serious problems.

Teens who are abused (or have been in the past) often have trouble sleeping, eating, and concentrating. They may not do well at school because they are angry or frightened, or feel like they just don't care anymore.

Many people who are abused distrust others. They may feel a lot of anger toward other people and themselves, and it can be hard to make friends. Abuse is a significant cause of depression in young people. Some teens can only feel better by doing things that could hurt them like cutting or abusing drugs or alcohol. They might even attempt suicide.

It's common for those who have been abused to feel upset, angry, and confused about what happened to them. They may feel guilty and embarrassed and blame themselves. But abuse is never the fault of the person who is being abused, no matter how much the abuser tries to blame others.

Abusers may manipulate somebody into keeping quiet by saying stuff like: "This is a secret between you and me," or "If you ever tell anybody, I'll hurt you or your mom," or "You're going to get in trouble if you tell. No one will believe you and you'll go to jail for lying." This is the abuser's way of making a person feel like nothing can be done so he or she won't report the abuse.

People who are abused might have trouble getting help because it means they'd be reporting on someone they love—someone who may be wonderful much of the time and awful to them only some of the time.

People might be afraid of the consequences of reporting abuse, either because they fear the abuser or the family is financially dependent on that person. For reasons like these, abuse often goes unreported and many kids and teens don't tell anyone what is going on.

# What Should Someone Who's Being Abused Do?

People who are being abused need to get help. Keeping the abuse a secret doesn't protect anyone from being abused—it only makes it more likely that the abuse will continue.

If you or anyone you know is being abused, talk to someone you or your friend can trust—a family member, a trusted teacher, a doctor, or a school or religious youth counselor. Many teachers and counselors have training in how to recognize and report abuse.

> Telephone and online directories list local child abuse and family violence hotline numbers that you can call for help. There's also Childhelp USA at (800) 4-A-CHILD ([800] 422-4453).

Sometimes people who are being abused by someone in their own home need to find a safe place to live temporarily. It is never easy to have to leave home, but it's sometimes necessary to be protected from further abuse. People who need to leave home to stay safe can find local shelters listed in the phone book or they can contact an abuse helpline. Sometimes a person can stay with a relative or friend.

People who are being abused often feel afraid, numb, or lonely. Getting help and support is an important first step toward feeling better.

Many teens who have experienced abuse find that painful emotions may linger even after the abuse stops. Working with a therapist is one way to sort through the complicated feelings and reactions that being abused creates, and the process can help to rebuild feelings of safety, confidence, and self-esteem.

# Chapter 2
# Emotional And Physical Abuse

## Verbal/Emotional Abuse

Verbal and emotional abuse can be hard to spot because there aren't physical signs. Emotional abuse happens when someone constantly yells at you or uses words to hurt you. Eventually, your self-esteem is damaged. Verbal and emotional abusers can be parents or other family members, a boyfriend, a girlfriend, a teacher, or anyone who makes you feel badly about yourself.

Someone who is an emotional abuser will use mean names, put-downs, insults, sexual harassment, or other ways to gain power over the other person.

## Signs Of Emotional Abuse

You may feel like if you're not being hurt physically, you are not being abused. But attempts to scare, isolate, or control you also are abuse. They can affect your physical and emotional well-being. And they often are a sign that physical abuse will follow.

You may be experiencing emotional abuse if someone:

- monitors what you're doing all the time

- unfairly accuses you of being unfaithful all the time

About This Chapter: Text under the heading "Verbal/Emotional Abuse" is excerpted from "Verbal/Emotional Abuse," Office on Women's Health (OWH), U.S. Department of Health and Human Services (HHS), September 22, 2009. Reviewed November 2016; Text under the heading "Signs Of Emotional Abuse" is excerpted from "Violence Against Women," Office on Women's Health (OWH), U.S. Department of Health and Human Services (HHS), September 30, 2015; remaining text is from "Physical Abuse," © 2016 Omnigraphics. Reviewed January 2016.

- prevents or discourages you from seeing friends or family

- tries to stop you from going to work or school

- gets angry in a way that is frightening to you

- controls how you spend your money

- humiliates you in front of others

- threatens to hurt you or people you care about

- threatens to harm himself or herself when upset with you

- says things like, "If I can't have you then no one can."

- decides things for you that you should decide (like what to wear or eat)

No one has the right to hurt you in any way.

# Physical Abuse

Physical abuse is any deliberate use of bodily force that causes pain, injury, or trauma to another person. Some examples of actions that are considered physical abuse include punching, hitting, slapping, smacking, kicking, scratching, biting, pinching, shaking, choking, burning, pulling hair, throwing objects, and forcing someone to swallow a harmful substance. Physical abuse can be perpetrated by anyone, including parents, siblings, other relatives, boyfriends, girlfriends, babysitters, other caregivers, and classmates.

In the case of parents and caregivers, corporal punishment or physical discipline that is applied to children in an excessive or inappropriate manner can be abusive. The risk of child abuse is highest among parents who are immature, lack parenting skills, do not understand developmentally appropriate behavior, and were not exposed to positive parental role models in their own childhood. Other factors related to physical abuse include financial stress or other crises in the home environment, and drug or alcohol addiction.

# Warning Signs And Negative Effects

The warning signs of physical abuse may be physical, emotional, or behavioral. Some of the possible physical indicators include bruises, cuts, abrasions, fractures, sprains, dislocations, burns, missing teeth, traumatic hair loss, internal injuries, and bleeding from body orifices. Since many types of physical injuries can result from accidents or participation in sports, it may be difficult to tell whether warning signs indicate abuse. Certain types of bruises are rarely accidental, however, including bilateral bruising on the arms, wrap-around bruising on the wrists, and bilateral bruising on the inner thighs.

In determining whether specific injuries are the result of physical abuse, it may be helpful to watch for patterns of similar injuries over time. Additional warning signs include injuries that are unexplained, explained in an implausible manner, or explained differently by various family members. Physical abuse may also be suspected if medical treatment is delayed or sought from several different practitioners to prevent any one doctor from noticing a pattern.

The emotional and behavioral signs of physical abuse vary widely, depending on the person. Some victims of physical abuse react by becoming angry, aggressive, or violent, while others respond by becoming extremely quiet, passive, and withdrawn. It is common for people who experience physical abuse to feel frightened, worried, sad, depressed, worthless, lonely, isolated, angry, frustrated, numb, or desperate. Victims may also have trouble sleeping, concentrating on tasks, or eating normally. They may consider running away from home or harming themselves. Although many people who are physically abused feel guilty and worry that they may have done something to deserve the mistreatment, it is important to understand that physical abuse is never the victim's fault.

Some of the effects of physical abuse may continue over the long term. Studies show that people who are physically abused as children are more likely to behave aggressively as teenagers and adults. In fact, up to one-third of children who experience physical abuse become abusers in adulthood. Abused children also face a much greater risk of substance abuse, depression, posttraumatic stress disorder, and suicide.

## Sources Of Help And Support

When physical abuse occurs regularly over a long time, the victim may begin to see it as a normal part of life. Some people who experience physical abuse may be confused because they still have feelings of love or affection for the person who is hurting them. If the abuser is a parent or caregiver, the victim may worry that stopping the abuse would mean being alone or being placed in foster care. No matter what the circumstances, however, physical abuse is always wrong, and there are many sources available to help make it stop.

The first step in stopping physical abuse is confiding in a trusted person. It is important to feel comfortable and safe with the person chosen, whether it is a parent, family member, neighbor, religious leader, teacher, counselor, school nurse, or coach. Since talking about physical abuse can be difficult, it may be helpful to start by putting the information in writing. There are also websites and hotlines available to provide resources and support for people trying to stop physical abuse.

Telling someone about physical abuse not only helps the victim, but it can also protect other people from being abused in the future. People in certain professions—including teachers, social workers, doctors, therapists, and day-care providers—who notice signs of child abuse are required by law to report it to law enforcement or child protective services agencies.

## References

1. Dubowitz, H. and D. DePanfilis, "What Is Physical Abuse?" Handbook for Child Protection Practice, Thousand Oaks, CA: Sage, 2000.

2. "Physical Abuse," ChildLine, n.d.

# Chapter 3
# Domestic Violence

## What Is Domestic Violence?

Domestic violence is defined as a pattern of abusive behavior in any relationship that is used by one partner to gain or maintain power and control over another intimate partner. Domestic violence can be physical, sexual, emotional, economic, or psychological actions or threats of actions that influence another person. This includes any behaviors that intimidate, manipulate, humiliate, isolate, frighten, terrorize, coerce, threaten, blame, hurt, injure, or wound someone.

**Physical Abuse:** Hitting, slapping, shoving, grabbing, pinching, biting, hair pulling, etc., are types of physical abuse. This type of abuse also includes denying a partner medical care or forcing alcohol and/or drug use upon him or her.

**Sexual Abuse:** Coercing or attempting to coerce any sexual contact or behavior without consent. Sexual abuse includes, but is certainly not limited to, marital rape, attacks on sexual parts of the body, forcing sex after physical violence has occurred, or treating one in a sexually demeaning manner.

**Emotional Abuse:** Undermining an individual's sense of self-worth and/or self-esteem is abusive. This may include, but is not limited to constant criticism, diminishing one's abilities, name-calling, or damaging one's relationship with his or her children.

---

About This Chapter: Text under the heading "What Is Domestic Violence?" is excerpted from "Domestic Violence," U.S. Department of Justice (DOJ), October 5, 2016; Text under the heading "What Is Intimate Partner Violence?" is excerpted from "Intimate Partner Violence," Centers for Disease Control and Prevention (CDC), July 20, 2016; Text beginning with the heading "Getting Help For Domestic Abuse" is excerpted from "Violence Against Women," Office on Women's Health (OWH), U.S. Department of Health and Human Services (HHS), September 30, 2015.

**Economic Abuse:** It is defined as making or attempting to make an individual financially dependent by maintaining total control over financial resources, withholding one's access to money, or forbidding one's attendance at school or employment.

**Psychological Abuse:** Elements of psychological abuse include—but are not limited to—causing fear by intimidation; threatening physical harm to self, partner, children, or partner's family or friends; destruction of pets and property; and forcing isolation from family, friends, or school and/or work.

Domestic violence can happen to anyone regardless of race, age, sexual orientation, religion, or gender. Domestic violence affects people of all socioeconomic backgrounds and education levels. Domestic violence occurs in both opposite-sex and same-sex relationships and can happen to intimate partners who are married, living together, or dating.

Domestic violence not only affects those who are abused, but also has a substantial effect on family members, friends, co-workers, other witnesses, and the community at large. Children, who grow up witnessing domestic violence, are among those seriously affected by this crime. Frequent exposure to violence in the home not only predisposes children to numerous social and physical problems, but also teaches them that violence is a normal way of life—therefore, increasing their risk of becoming society's next generation of victims and abusers.

## Key Points About Domestic Violence

- If you are in immediate danger, you can call 911.
- Often, abuse starts as emotional abuse and then becomes physical later.
- Sometimes it is hard to know if you are being abused.
- An abusive partner may try to make you feel like the abuse is your fault.
- Violence can cause serious physical and emotional problems, including depression and posttraumatic stress disorder.
- There probably will be times when the abuser is very kind.
- An abusive partner needs to get help from a mental health professional.

Being hurt by someone close to you is awful. Reach out for support from family, friends, and community organizations.

*Source: "Violence Against Women," Office on Women's Health (OWH), U.S. Department of Health and Human Services (HHS), September 30, 2015.*

# What Is Intimate Partner Violence?

Intimate partner violence (IPV) is a serious, preventable public health problem that affects millions of Americans. The term "intimate partner violence" describes physical violence, sexual violence, stalking and psychological aggression (including coercive acts) by a current or former intimate partner.

An intimate partner is a person with whom one has a close personal relationship that can be characterized by the following:

- Emotional connectedness

- Regular contact

- Ongoing physical contact and/or sexual behavior

- Identity as a couple

- Familiarity and knowledge about each other's lives

The relationship need not involve all of these dimensions. Examples of intimate partners include current or former spouses, boyfriends or girlfriends, dating partners, or sexual partners. IPV can occur between heterosexual or same-sex couples and does not require sexual intimacy.

IPV can vary in frequency and severity. It occurs on a continuum, ranging from one episode that might or might not have lasting impact to chronic and severe episodes over a period of years.

There are four main types of IPV.

- **Physical violence** is the intentional use of physical force with the potential for causing death, disability, injury, or harm. Physical violence includes, but is not limited to, scratching; pushing; shoving; throwing; grabbing; biting; choking; shaking; aggressive hair pulling; slapping; punching; hitting; burning; use of a weapon; and use of restraints or one's body, size, or strength against another person. Physical violence also includes coercing other people to commit any of the above acts.

- **Sexual violence** is divided into five categories. Any of these acts constitute sexual violence, whether attempted or completed. Additionally all of these acts occur without the victim's freely given consent, including cases in which the victim is unable to consent due to being too intoxicated (e.g., incapacitation, lack of consciousness, or lack of awareness) through their voluntary or involuntary use of alcohol or drugs.

- **Rape or penetration of victim**—This includes completed or attempted, forced or alcohol/drug-facilitated unwanted vaginal, oral, or anal insertion. Forced penetration occurs through the perpetrator's use of physical force against the victim or threats to physically harm the victim.

- **Victim was made to penetrate someone else**—This includes completed or attempted, forced or alcohol/drug-facilitated incidents when the victim was made to sexually penetrate a perpetrator or someone else without the victim's consent.

- **Non-physically pressured unwanted penetration**—This includes incidents in which the victim was pressured verbally or through intimidation or misuse of authority to consent or acquiesce to being penetrated.

- **Unwanted sexual contact**—This includes intentional touching of the victim or making the victim touch the perpetrator, either directly or through the clothing, on the genitalia, anus, groin, breast, inner thigh, or buttocks without the victim's consent

- **Non-contact unwanted sexual experiences**—This includes unwanted sexual events that are not of a physical nature that occur without the victim's consent. Examples include unwanted exposure to sexual situations (e.g., pornography); verbal or behavioral sexual harassment; threats of sexual violence to accomplish some other end; and / or unwanted filming, taking or disseminating photographs of a sexual nature of another person.

- **Stalking** is a pattern of repeated, unwanted, attention and contact that causes fear or concern for one's own safety or the safety of someone else (e.g., family member or friend). Some examples include repeated, unwanted phone calls, emails, or texts; leaving cards, letters, flowers, or other items when the victim does not want them; watching or following from a distance; spying; approaching or showing up in places when the victim does not want to see them; sneaking into the victim's home or car; damaging the victim's personal property; harming or threatening the victim's pet; and making threats to physically harm the victim.

- **Psychological Aggression** is the use of verbal and non-verbal communication with the intent to harm another person mentally or emotionally, and/or to exert control over another person. Psychological aggression can include expressive aggression (e.g., name-calling, humiliating); coercive control (e.g., limiting access to transportation, money, friends, and family; excessive monitoring of whereabouts); threats of physical or sexual violence; control of reproductive or sexual health (e.g., refusal to use birth control; coerced pregnancy termination); exploitation of victim's vulnerability (e.g., immigration status, disability); exploitation of perpetrator's vulnerability; and presenting false information to the victim with the intent of making them doubt their own memory or perception (e.g., mind games).

# Getting Help For Domestic Abuse

If you are being abused, get help. The longer the abuse goes on, the more damage it can cause. You are not alone. There are people who will believe you and who want to help.

Consider these steps if you are in an abusive situation:

- If you are in immediate danger, call 911 or leave.

- If you are hurt, go to a local hospital emergency room.

- Call the National Domestic Violence Hotline at 800-799-SAFE (800-799-7233) or 800-787-3224 (TDD). The hotline offers help in many languages 24 hours a day, every day. Hotline staff can give you the phone numbers of local shelters and other resources.

- Plan ahead. Violence sometimes gets worse right after leaving, so think about a safe place to go. You can get advice from the National Domestic Violence Hotline.

- Look up state resources for a list of local places to get help.

- Review a full checklist of items to take if you leave, such as your marriage license, any children's birth certificates, and money. Put these things somewhere you can get them quickly. Of course, if you are in immediate danger, leave without them.

- Have a cellphone handy. Try not to call for help from your home phone or a shared cellphone since an abuser may be able to trace the numbers. If possible, get a prepaid cellphone or your own cellphone. Some domestic violence shelters offer free cellphones.

- Contact your family court (or domestic violence court, if offered by your state) for information about getting a court order of protection. If you need legal help but don't have much money, your local domestic violence agency may be able to help you find a lawyer who will work for free.

- Create a code word to use with friends and family to let them know you are in danger. If possible, agree on a secret location where they can pick you up.

- If you can, hide an extra set of car keys so you can leave if your partner takes away your keys.

- When you leave, try to bring any evidence of abuse, like threatening notes from your partner or copies of police reports.

- Reach out to someone you trust—a family member, friend, co-worker, or spiritual leader. Look into ways to get emotional help, like a support group or mental health professional.

Sometimes a woman may hit a man first, and then she ends up getting hurt badly because the man is stronger. Talk to your doctor or a mental health professional if you sometimes hit or use other kinds of violence.

# Transitional Housing

Transitional housing focuses on giving families a safe space and time to recover from domestic violence. Families live independently, in separate apartments, while they also receive needed services. Services can include:

- Individual counseling

- Family counseling

- Support groups

- Job training

- Help finding affordable, permanent housing

- Legal help

- Childcare and others services for your children

# Domestic Abuse And HIV

Domestic violence and HIV are connected in a number of ways:

- **If you are currently in an abusive relationship, you are more likely to get HIV.** That's partly because abusive men are more likely to have sexual partners other than their wife. Also, if you are in an abusive relationship, your partner may force you to have sex, and forced sex can cause cuts that can let HIV enter your body. In addition, an abusive partner may refuse to use a condom, which could put you at risk for HIV.

- **If you are physically or sexually abused as a child, you may have an increased risk of getting HIV.** That's because women who were abused as children are more likely to have a higher number of sex partners. Women who were abused as children are also less likely to use condoms each time they have sex.

- **Women with HIV may be at risk of violence when they tell a partner about their HIV status.** Take these steps to lower the risk that your partner will react violently:

  - Tell your partner that you have HIV **before** you get sexually involved.

  - Tell your partner that you have HIV in a semi-public place. A public park is a good place, because it gives you some privacy, but other people are around in case you need help.

  - If you feel **at all** threatened by your partner's reaction, stop seeing each other or at least keep meetings public for a while.

# Chapter 4
# Child Abuse

## What Is Child Abuse And Neglect?

Child abuse and neglect is any act or series of acts of commission or omission by a parent or other caregiver (e.g., clergy, coach, teacher) that results in harm, potential for harm, or threat of harm to a child.

### Acts Of Commission (Child Abuse)

Words or overt actions that cause harm, potential harm, or threat of harm

Acts of commission are deliberate and intentional; however, harm to a child might not be the intended consequence. Intention only applies to caregiver acts—not the consequences of those acts. For example, a caregiver might intend to hit a child as punishment (i.e., hitting the child is not accidental or unintentional), but not intend to cause the child to have a concussion. The following types of maltreatment involve acts of commission:

- Physical abuse

- Sexual abuse

- Psychological abuse

### Acts Of Omission (Child Neglect)

Failure to provide needs or to protect from harm or potential harm

Acts of omission are the failure to provide for a child's basic physical, emotional, or educational needs or to protect a child from harm or potential harm. Like acts of commission, harm

About This Chapter: This chapter includes text excerpted from "Child Maltreatment," Centers for Disease Control and Prevention (CDC), March 28, 2016.

to a child might not be the intended consequence. The following types of maltreatment involve acts of omission:

- Physical neglect

- Emotional neglect

- Medical and dental neglect

- Educational neglect

- Inadequate supervision

- Exposure to violent environments

# Risk And Protective Factors

A combination of individual, relational, community, and societal factors contribute to the risk of child abuse and neglect. Although children are not responsible for the harm inflicted upon them, certain characteristics have been found to increase their risk of being maltreated. Risk factors are those characteristics associated with child abuse and neglect—they may or may not be direct causes.

## Risk Factors For Victimization

### Individual Risk Factors

- Children younger than 4 years of age

- Special needs that may increase caregiver burden (e.g., disabilities, mental retardation, mental health issues, and chronic physical illnesses)

## Risk Factors For Perpetration

### Individual Risk Factors

- Parents' lack of understanding of children's needs, child development and parenting skills

- Parents' history of child maltreatment in family of origin

- Substance abuse and/or mental health issues including depression in the family

- Parental characteristics such as young age, low education, single parenthood, large number of dependent children, and low income

- Nonbiological, transient caregivers in the home (e.g., mother's male partner)
- Parental thoughts and emotions that tend to support or justify maltreatment behaviors

## Family Risk Factors

- Social isolation
- Family disorganization, dissolution, and violence, including intimate partner violence
- Parenting stress, poor parent-child relationships, and negative interactions

## Community Risk Factors

- Community violence
- Concentrated neighborhood disadvantage (e.g., high poverty and residential instability, high unemployment rates, and high density of alcohol outlets), and poor social connections.

# Protective Factors For Child Maltreatment

Protective factors buffer children from being abused or neglected. These factors exist at various levels. Protective factors have not been studied as extensively or rigorously as risk factors. However, identifying and understanding protective factors are equally as important as researching risk factors.

There is scientific evidence to support the following protective factor:

## Family Protective Factors

Supportive family environment and social networks

Several other potential protective factors have been identified. Research is ongoing to determine whether the following factors do indeed buffer children from maltreatment.

### Family Protective Factors

- Nurturing parenting skills
- Stable family relationships
- Household rules and child monitoring
- Parental employment

- Adequate housing

- Access to healthcare and social services

- Caring adults outside the family who can serve as role models or mentors

## Community Protective Factors

Communities that support parents and take responsibility for preventing abuse

# Chapter 5

# Children Of Addicted Parents: Increased Risks

## The Relationship Between Substance Use Disorders And Child Maltreatment

It is difficult to provide precise, current statistics on the number of families in child welfare affected by parental substance use or dependency since there is no ongoing, standardized, national data collection on the topic. In a 1999 report to Congress, the U.S. Department of Health and Human Services (HHS) reported that studies showed that between one-third and two-thirds of child maltreatment cases were affected by substance use to some degree. More recent research reviews suggest that the range may be even wider. The variation in estimates may be attributable, in part, to differences in the populations studied and the type of child welfare involvement (e.g., reports, substantiation, out-of-home placement); differences in how substance use (or substance abuse or substance use disorder) is defined and measured; and variations in State and local child welfare policies and practices for case documentation of substance abuse.

## Parental Substance Abuse As A Risk Factor For Maltreatment And Child Welfare Involvement

Parental substance abuse is recognized as a risk factor for child maltreatment and child welfare involvement. Research shows that children with parents who abuse alcohol or drugs are more likely to experience abuse or neglect than children in other households. One longitudinal study identified parental substance abuse (specifically, maternal drug use) as one of

About This Chapter: This chapter includes text excerpted from "Parental Substance Use And The Child Welfare System," Child Welfare Information Gateway, U.S. Department of Health and Human Services (HHS), October 2014.

five key factors that predicted a report to child protective services (CPS) for abuse or neglect. Once a report is substantiated, children of parents with substance use issues are more likely to be placed in out-of-home care and more likely to stay in care longer than other children. The National Survey of Child and Adolescent Well-Being (NSCAW) estimates that 61 percent of infants and 41 percent of older children in out of-home care are from families with active alcohol or drug abuse.

According to data in the Adoption and Foster Care Analysis and Reporting System (AFCARS), parental substance abuse is frequently reported as a reason for removal, particularly in combination with neglect. For almost 31 percent of all children placed in foster care in 2012, parental alcohol or drug use was the documented reason for removal, and in several States that percentage surpassed 60 percent. Nevertheless, many caregivers whose children remain at home after an investigation also have substance abuse issues. NSCAW found that the need for substance abuse services among in-home caregivers receiving child welfare services was substantially higher than that of adults nationwide (29 percent as compared with 20 percent, respectively, for parents ages 18 to 25, and 29 percent versus 7 percent for parents over age 26).

## Role Of Co-occurring Issues

While the link between substance abuse and child maltreatment is well documented, it is not clear how much is a direct causal connection and how much can be attributed to other co-occurring issues. National data reveal that slightly more than one-third of adults with substance use disorders have a co-occurring mental illness. Research on women with substance abuse problems shows high rates of posttraumatic stress disorder (PTSD), most commonly stemming from a history of childhood physical and/ or sexual assault. Many parents with substance abuse problems also experience social isolation, poverty, unstable housing, and domestic violence. These co-occurring issues may contribute to both the substance use and the child maltreatment. Evidence increasingly points to a critical role of stress and reactions within the brain to stress, which can lead to both drug-seeking activity and inappropriate caregiving.

# Impact Of Parental Substance Use On Children

The way parents with substance use disorders behave and interact with their children can have a multifaceted impact on the children. The effects can be both indirect (e.g., through a chaotic living environment) and direct (e.g., physical or sexual abuse). Parental substance use can affect parenting, prenatal development, and early childhood and adolescent development.

It is important to recognize, however, that not all children of parents with substance use issues will suffer abuse, neglect, or other negative outcomes.

## Parenting

A parent's substance use disorder may affect his or her ability to function effectively in a parental role. Ineffective or inconsistent parenting can be due to the following:

- physical or mental impairments caused by alcohol or other drugs
- reduced capacity to respond to a child's cues and needs
- difficulties regulating emotions and controlling anger and impulsivity
- disruptions in healthy parent-child attachment
- spending limited funds on alcohol and drugs rather than food or other household needs
- spending time seeking out, manufacturing, or using alcohol or other drugs
- incarceration, which can result in inadequate or inappropriate supervision for children
- estrangement from family and other social supports

Family life for children with one or both parents that abuse drugs or alcohol often can be chaotic and unpredictable. Children's basic needs—including nutrition, supervision, and nurturing—may go unmet, which can result in neglect. These families often experience a number of other problems—such as mental illness, domestic violence, unemployment, and housing instability—that also affect parenting and contribute to high levels of stress. A parent with a substance abuse disorder may be unable to regulate stress and other emotions, which can lead to impulsive and reactive behavior that may escalate to physical abuse.

Different substances may have different effects on parenting and safety. For example, the threats to a child of a parent who becomes sedated and inattentive after drinking excessively differ from the threats posed by a parent who exhibits aggressive side effects from methamphetamine use. Dangers may be posed not only from use of illegal drugs, but also, and increasingly, from abuse of prescription drugs (pain relievers, anti-anxiety medicines, and sleeping pills).

Polysubstance use (multiple drugs) may make it difficult to determine the specific and compounded effects on any individual. Further, risks for the child's safety may differ depending upon the level and severity of parental substance use and associated adverse effects.

## Prenatal And Infant Development

The effects of parental substance use disorders on a child can begin before the child is born. Maternal drug and alcohol use during pregnancy have been associated with premature birth, low birth weight, slowed growth, and a variety of physical, emotional, behavioral, and cognitive problems. Research suggests powerful effects of legal drugs, such as tobacco, as well as illegal drugs on prenatal and early childhood development.

Fetal alcohol spectrum disorders (FASD) are a set of conditions that affect an estimated 40,000 infants born each year to mothers who drank alcohol during pregnancy. Children with FASD may experience mild to severe physical, mental, behavioral, and/or learning disabilities, some of which may have lifelong implications (e.g., brain damage, physical defects, attention deficits). In addition, increasing numbers of newborns—approximately 3 per 1,000 hospital births each year—are affected by neonatal abstinence syndrome (NAS), a group of problems that occur in a newborn who was exposed prenatally to addictive illegal or prescription drugs.

The full impact of prenatal substance exposure depends on a number of factors. These include the frequency, timing, and type of substances used by pregnant women; co-occurring environmental deficiencies; and the extent of prenatal care. Research suggests that some of the negative outcomes of prenatal exposure can be improved by supportive home environments and positive parenting practices.

## Child And Adolescent Development

Children and youth of parents who use or abuse substances and have parenting difficulties have an increased chance of experiencing a variety of negative outcomes:

- poor cognitive, social, and emotional development
- depression, anxiety, and other trauma and mental health symptoms
- physical and health issues
- substance use problems

Parental substance use can affect the well-being of children and youth in complex ways. For example, an infant who receives inconsistent care and nurturing from a parent engaged in addiction-related behaviors may suffer from attachment difficulties that can then interfere with the growing child's emotional development. Adolescent children of parents with substance use disorders, particularly those who have experienced child maltreatment and foster care, may turn to substances themselves as a coping mechanism. In addition, children of parents with substance use issues are more likely to experience trauma and its effects, which include difficulties with concentration and learning, controlling physical and emotional responses to stress, and forming trusting relationships.

# Child Welfare Laws Related To Parental Substance Use

In response to concerns over the potential negative impact on children of parental substance abuse and illegal drug-related activities, approximately 47 States and the District of Columbia have child protection laws that address some aspect of parental substance use. Some States have expanded their civil definitions of child abuse and neglect to include a caregiver's use of a controlled substance that impairs the ability to adequately care for a child and/or exposure of a child to illegal drug activity (e.g., sale or distribution of drugs, home-based meth labs). Exposure of children to illegal drug activity is also addressed in 33 States' criminal statutes.

Federal and State laws also address prenatal drug exposure. The Child Abuse Prevention and Treatment Act (CAPTA) requires States receiving CAPTA funds to have policies and procedures for healthcare personnel to notify CPS of substance-exposed newborns and to develop procedures for safe care of affected infants. As yet, there are no national data on CAPTA-related reports for substance-exposed newborns. In some State statutes, substance abuse during pregnancy is considered child abuse and/or grounds for termination of parental rights. State statutes and State and local policies vary widely in their requirements for reporting suspected prenatal drug abuse, testing for drug exposure, CPS response, forced admission to treatment of pregnant women who use drugs, and priority access for pregnant women to State funded treatment programs.

# Innovative Prevention And Treatment Approaches

While parental substance abuse continues to be a major challenge in child welfare, the past two decades have witnessed some new and more effective approaches and innovative programs to address child protection for families where substance abuse is an issue. Some examples of promising and innovative prevention and treatment approaches include the following:

- Promotion of protective factors, such as social connections, concrete supports, and parenting knowledge, to support families and buffer risks.

- Early identification of at-risk families in substance abuse treatment programs and through expanded prenatal screening initiatives so that prevention services can be provided to promote child safety and well-being in the home.

- Priority and timely access to substance abuse treatment slots for mothers involved in the child welfare system.

- Gender-sensitive treatment and support services that respond to the specific needs, characteristics, and co-occurring issues of women who have substance use disorders.

- Family-centered treatment services, including inpatient treatment for mothers in facilities where they can have their children with them and programs that provide services to each family member.

- Recovery coaches or mentoring of parents to support treatment, recovery, and parenting.

- Shared family care in which a family experiencing parental substance use and child maltreatment is placed with a host family for support and mentoring.

# Chapter 6
# Elder Abuse

## What Is Elder Abuse?

Elder abuse is an intentional act, or failure to act, by a caregiver or another person in a relationship involving an expectation of trust that causes or creates a risk of harm to an older adult. (An older adult is defined as someone age 60 or older.) Forms of elder abuse are below.

- **Physical Abuse:** the intentional use of physical force that results in acute or chronic illness, bodily injury, physical pain, functional impairment, distress, or death. Physical abuse may include, but is not limited to, violent acts such as striking (with or without an object or weapon), hitting, beating, scratching, biting, choking, suffocation, pushing, shoving, shaking, slapping, kicking, stomping, pinching, and burning.

- **Sexual Abuse or Abusive Sexual Contact:** forced or unwanted sexual interaction (touching and non-touching acts) of any kind with an older adult. This may include, but is not limited to, forced or unwanted completed or attempted contact between the penis and the vulva or the penis and the anus involving penetration, however slight; forced or unwanted contact between the mouth and the penis, vulva, or anus; forced or unwanted penetration of the anal or genital opening of another person by a hand, finger, or other object; forced or unwanted intentional touching, either directly or through the clothing, of the genitalia, anus, groin, breast, inner thigh, or buttocks. These acts also qualify as sexual abuse if they are committed against an incapacitated person who is not competent to give informed approval.

About This Chapter: This chapter includes text excerpted from "Elder Abuse," Centers for Disease Control and Prevention (CDC), January 14, 2014.

- **Emotional or Psychological Abuse:** verbal or nonverbal behavior that results in the infliction of anguish, mental pain, fear, or distress. Examples of tactics that may exemplify Emotional or Psychological Abuse include behaviors intended to humiliate (e.g., calling names or insults), threaten (e.g., expressing an intent to initiate nursing home placement), isolate (e.g., seclusion from family and friends), or control (e.g., prohibiting or limiting access to transportation, telephone, money or other resources) an older adult).

- **Neglect:** failure by a caregiver or other responsible person to protect an elder from harm, or the failure to meet needs for essential medical care, nutrition, hydration, hygiene, clothing, basic activities of daily living or shelter, which results in a serious risk of compromised health and safety. Examples include not providing adequate nutrition, hygiene, clothing, shelter, or access to necessary healthcare; or failure to prevent exposure to unsafe activities and environments.

- **Financial Abuse or Exploitation:** the illegal, unauthorized, or improper use of an older individual's resources by a caregiver or other person in a trusting relationship, for the benefit of someone other than the older individual. This includes, but is not limited to, depriving an older person of rightful access to, information about, or use of, personal benefits, resources, belongings, or assets. Examples include forgery, misuse or theft of money or possessions; use of coercion or deception to surrender finances or property; or improper use of guardianship or power of attorney.

# Risk And Protective Factors

## Risk Factors

A combination of individual, relational, community, and societal factors contribute to the risk of becoming a perpetrator of elder abuse. They are contributing factors and may or may not be direct causes.

Understanding these factors can help identify various opportunities for prevention.

### Risk Factors For Perpetration

**Individual Level**

- Current diagnosis of mental illness
- Current abuse of alcohol
- High levels of hostility

- Poor or inadequate preparation or training for care giving responsibilities

- Assumption of caregiving responsibilities at an early age

- Inadequate coping skills

- Exposure to abuse as a child

**Relationship Level**

- High financial and emotional dependence upon a vulnerable elder

- Past experience of disruptive behavior

- Lack of social support

- Lack of formal support

**Community Level**

Formal services, such as respite care for those providing care to elders, are limited, inaccessible, or unavailable

**Societal Level**

A culture where:

- there is high tolerance and acceptance of aggressive behavior;

- healthcare personnel, guardians, and other agents are given greater freedom in routine care provision and decision making;

- family members are expected to care for elders without seeking help from others;

- persons are encouraged to endure suffering or remain silent regarding their pains; or

- there are negative beliefs about aging and elders.

In addition to the above factors, there are also specific characteristics of institutional settings that may increase the risk for perpetration of vulnerable elders in these settings, including: unsympathetic or negative attitudes toward residents, chronic staffing problems, lack of administrative oversight, staff burnout, and stressful working conditions.

## Protective Factors for Elder Abuse

Protective factors reduce risk for perpetrating abuse and neglect. Protective factors have not been studied as extensively or rigorously as risk factors. However, identifying and understanding protective factors are equally as important as researching risk factors.

Several potential protective factors are identified below. Research is needed to determine whether these factors do indeed buffer elders from abuse.

## Protective Factors For Perpetration

**Relationship Level**

Having numerous, strong relationships with people of varying social status

**Community Level**

- Coordination of resources and services among community agencies and organizations that serve the elderly population and their caregivers.

- Higher levels of community cohesion and a strong sense of community or community identity

- Higher levels of community functionality and greater collective efficacy

Factors within institutional settings that may be protective include: effective monitoring systems in place; solid institutional policies and procedures regarding patient care; regular training on elder abuse and neglect for employees; education about and clear guidance on how durable power of attorney is to be used; and regular visits by family members, volunteers, and social workers.

# Consequences

## Prevalence Of Elder Abuse

Elder abuse, including neglect and exploitation, is experienced by one out of every ten people ages 60 and older who lives at home.

For every one case of elder abuse that is detected or reported, it is estimated that approximately 23 cases remain hidden.

## Consequences Of Elder Abuse

The possible physical and psychosocial consequences of elder abuse are numerous and varied. Few studies have examined the consequences of elder abuse and distinguished them from those linked to normal aging.

## Physical Effects

The most immediate probable physical effects include the following:

- Welts, wounds, and injuries (e.g., bruises, lacerations, dental problems, head injuries, broken bones, pressure sores)

- Persistent physical pain and soreness

- Nutrition and hydration issues

- Sleep disturbances

- Increased susceptibility to new illnesses (including sexually transmitted diseases)

- Exacerbation of preexisting health conditions

- Increased risks for premature death

## Psychological Effects

Established psychological effects of elder abuse include high levels of distress and depression.

Other potential psychological consequences that need further scientific study are

- Increased risks for developing fear and anxiety reactions

- Learned helplessness

- Posttraumatic stress disorder

# Prevention Strategies

Elder abuse is a serious problem that can have harmful effects on victims. The goal for elder abuse prevention is simple: to stop it from happening in the first place. However, the solutions are as complex as the problem.

Knowledge about what works to prevent elder abuse is growing. However, most prevention strategies and practices have not yet been rigorously evaluated to determine their effectiveness.

# Chapter 7
# Sibling Abuse

## Prevalence Of Sibling Abuse

The term "siblings" generally refers to biological brothers and sisters—children who share the same two parents—but in a broader sense it may also refer to any children who are part of a family unit. These include half siblings, who share one common parent, and step siblings, who are not biologically related but who become part of a family as a result of marriage or partnership between their parents. Studies have shown that the risk of sexual abuse is usually more common between step siblings, but accurate statistics are difficult to compile about abuse between related individuals because of the powerful societal taboo against incest, which causes it to go underreported due to embarrassment, fear, denial, or lack of understanding.

---

### Defining Sibling Abuse

When a child is victimized by a sibling, it is termed sibling abuse. Physical aggression—pushing, shoving, or more serious acts of violence—as well as bullying or harassment, are examples of sibling abuse. Unless serious physical harm takes place, parents may ignore this behavior, believing it to be normal childhood activity. But sibling abuse can have severe consequences for survivors, often troubling them well into adulthood.

---

## Classification Of Sibling Abuse

Sibling abuse is a fairly broad term that can be classified into three types:

- Physical sibling abuse

---

"Sibling Abuse," © 2016 Omnigraphics. Reviewed May 2016.

- Emotional or psychological sibling abuse

- Sexual sibling abuse

**Physical sibling abuse.** This is a very common form of sibling abuse, as arguments can often lead to physical fighting, pinching, slapping, or hair pulling. These conflicts may become abusive in the course of time and may escalate into violence or serious injury. Weapons, if used, may even result in fatal consequences. What begins as sibling rivalry, if not checked, may end up in tragedy within the family. One of the characteristic features of physical sibling abuse is that the perpetrator of the abuse is usually bigger and/or stronger than the victim, although this is not always the case. Physical sibling abuse is not gender-specific, and therefore children of either sex may be the abusers.

**Emotional/psychological sibling abuse.** Physical sibling abuse is often quite evident, making it somewhat easier to take steps to protect the victim. However, emotional or psychological sibling abuse can be harder to detect. It is also very difficult to measure the impact of this form of sibling abuse. Quarrels between the adults in the family or acts of bullying at school can leave a deep impression upon the young mind. A child may also be emotionally abused by acts like belittling, demeaning, frightening, humiliating, name-calling, or threatening. Survivors of such abuse may become emotionally closed off, withdrawing from social contact and preferring to be alone. They tend to underperform both at school and at home and to become aggressive in other areas of their lives. Identifying emotional abuse early can help head off future problems.

**Sexual sibling abuse.** Many types of sexual contact or related activity between siblings can be termed sexual sibling abuse. This can include such acts as using sexually toned language, exposing genitals to another sibling, inappropriate touching, deliberate exposure to pornography, and sexual assaults or rape. Sexual sibling abuse can occur between full siblings, half siblings, or step siblings, although it is generally more common in the case of a half sibling or step sibling. The general belief is that boys tend to be the perpetrators, but there is also considerable evidence of girls being abusers.

# Risk Factors For Sibling Abuse

There are several factors that may increase the likelihood of sibling abuse, and it is vital that parents understand the root cause behind such behavior. Some factors that researchers have identified include:

- parents absent from the home for long periods of time

- lack of emotional attachment between parents and children

- parents allowing sibling rivalry and fights to go unchecked

- parents' inability to teach their children to deal with conflicts in a healthy manner

- parents not intervening when children are involved in violent acts

- parents creating a competitive environment by favoritism or frequently comparing siblings to each other

- denial of the problem's existence, both by parents and children

- overburdening children by giving responsibilities beyond their ability

- exposure to violence from different environments, such as home, media, and school

- parents failing to teach their children about sexuality and their personal safety

- children who witness to, or are victims of, sexual abuse

- early access to pornography

# Detecting Sibling Abuse

Sibling abuse may often be difficult to detect, especially when both parents are busy with their professional lives. Parents need to be alert to identify this behavior and take necessary action as early as possible. One symptom of sibling abuse is when one child is almost always the aggressor, while the other tends to be the victim. Other signs of sibling abuse include:

- a child avoids his or her sibling

- noticeable changes in behavior, eating habits, and sleep patterns

- frequent nightmares

- a child stages abuse in a play or reveals it in a story

- a child acts out in an inappropriate sexual manner

- increase in the intensity of animosity between the siblings

# Safeguarding Children From Sibling Abuse

Some steps that parents can take to help safeguard children from sibling abuse include:

- Discourage rivalry between siblings.

- Establish rules that will bar children from indulging in emotional abuse of their siblings, and stick to them so that children realize their importance.

- Give responsibilities to children based on their abilities, rather than overburdening them with tasks for which they are unprepared.

- Talk to children on a regular basis to gain their trust, and encourage them to ask for help from parents when they need it.

- Learn the art of mediating conflicts.

- Teach children that any kind of unwanted physical contact is inappropriate and should be reported to an adult.

- Build a healthy environment for sharing and talking about any issues, especially sexual issues.

- Be aware of children's media preferences to identify inappropriate videos, games, music, etc.

# Dealing With Sibling Abuse

Acts like biting, hitting, or physical torture of a child by his or her sibling should not be taken lightly. Parents need to intervene and take necessary actions, including:

- Separate the siblings whenever they indulge in any kind of violence.

- When the situation is under control, discuss the behavior with all the members of the family, as well as the children involved.

- Listen patiently to understand the children's feelings.

- Restate what they say to clarify your understanding of the problem.

- Encourage the children to work together.

- Do not ignore, blame, or punish the child, but take a neutral stand and avoid favoritism.

- Be sure the children know the family rules, as well as the consequences of failing to follow them.

- Teach the children anger management techniques.

- Follow up by observing future behavior carefully.

- Seek professional help if the parents feel that things are beyond their control.

# Sibling Abuse And Its Impact In Later Life

Events or incidents of sibling abuse that take place during childhood may have long-term psychological effects whose impact may not be revealed until a later stage of life. Researchers have found that these effects may include:

- alcohol and drug addiction

- anxiety

- depression

- eating disorders

- lack of trust

- low self-esteem

# Conclusion

Children who have been victims of sibling abuse tend to have feelings of insecurity and poor self-image well into adulthood. As much as physical abuse, emotional sibling abuse has a long-lasting impact. And the effects of this behavior do not only affect the victim. The abuser, too, has the potential to indulge in abusive relationships throughout his or her adulthood, making intervention critical for both individuals.

## References

1. "Sibling Abuse Help Guide," LeavingAbuse, August 23, 2015.

2. Boyse RN, Kyla. "Sibling Abuse," University of Michigan Health System, November 2012.

# Chapter 8
# Sexual Abuse of Women

## What Is Sexual Assault?[1]

Sexual assault is defined as any sort of sexual activity between two or more people in which one of the people is involved against her will.

The sexual activity involved in an assault can include many different experiences. Women can be the victims of unwanted touching, grabbing, oral sex, anal sex, sexual penetration with an object, and/or sexual intercourse.

There are a lot of ways that women can be involved in sexual activity against their will. The force used by the aggressor can be either physical or non-physical. Some examples of how women are forced or pressured into having sex include being:

- taken advantage of by someone who has some form of authority over them (for example doctor, teacher, boss)

- bribed or manipulated into sexual activity against her will

- unable to give her consent because she is under the influence of alcohol or drugs

- threatened to be hurt or that people that she cares about will be hurt

- physically forced or violently assaulted

---

About This Chapter: This chapter contains text excerpted from documents published by two public domain sources. Text under headings marked 1 are excerpted from "Sexual Assault Against Females," U.S. Department of Veterans Affairs (VA), August 13, 2015; Text under heading marked 2 are excerpted from "Violence Against Women," Office on Women's Health (OWH), U.S. Department of Health and Human Services (HHS), July 16, 2012. Reviewed November 2016.

# Who Commits Sexual Assaults?

Often, when we think about who commits sexual assault or rape, we imagine the aggressor is a stranger to the victim. Contrary to popular belief, sexual assault does not typically occur between strangers. The National Crime Victimization Survey (NCVS), conducted by the U.S. Department of Justice (DOJ), found that about four of every five sexually assaulted women were attacked by a current or former husband, cohabitating partner, friend, or date. Strangers committed only about one of every five of the assaults that were reported in the survey.

# How Often Do Sexual Assaults Happen?

Estimating rates of sexual violence against women is a difficult task. Many factors stop women from reporting these crimes to police and to interviewers collecting statistics on the rate of crime in our country. Women may not want to report that they were assaulted because it is such a personal experience, because they blame themselves, because they are afraid of how others may react, and because they do not think it is useful to make such a report. However, there are statistics that show sexual assault is a problem in our country. For example, a large-scale study conducted on several college campuses found that one of every five women reported that they had been raped in their lifetime.

# Types Of Violence Against Women[2]

Violence strikes women from all kinds of backgrounds and of all ages. It can happen at work, on the street, or at home. It has different types of violence and ways to stay safe.

- Dating violence
- Domestic and intimate partner violence
- Emotional abuse
- Human trafficking
- Same-sex relationship violence
- Sexual assault and abuse
- Stalking
- Violence against immigrant and refugee women
- Violence against women at work
- Violence against women with disabilities

Sometimes, women are attacked by strangers, but most often they are hurt by people who are close to them, such as a husband or partner. Whether you are attacked by a stranger or mistreated by a partner, violence and abuse can have terrible effects.

# What Happens To Women After They Are Sexually Assaulted?[1]

After a sexual assault, women can experience a wide range of reactions. It is very important to note that there is no single pattern of response. Some women respond immediately, others may have delayed reactions. Some women are affected by the assault for a long time, but others appear to recover more quickly.

In the time just after a sexual assault, many women report feeling shock, confusion, anxiety, and/or numbness. Sometimes women will experience feelings of denial. In other words, they may not fully accept what has happened to them or they may downplay the intensity of the experience. This reaction may be more common among women who are assaulted by someone they know.

# What Are Some Early Reactions To Sexual Assault?

In the first few days and weeks following the assault, it is very normal for a woman to experience intense and sometimes unpredictable emotions. She may have repeated strong memories of the event that are difficult to ignore, and nightmares are not uncommon. Women also report having difficulty concentrating and sleeping, and they may feel jumpy or on edge. While these initial reactions are normal and expected, some women may have severe, highly disruptive symptoms that make it very difficult to function in the first month following the assault.

# What Are Some Other Reactions That Women Have Following A Sexual Assault?

## Major Depressive Disorder (MDD)

Depression is a common reaction following sexual assault. Symptoms of MDD can include a depressed mood, an inability to enjoy things, difficulty sleeping, changes in patterns of sleeping and eating, problems in concentration and decision-making, feelings of guilt, hopelessness, and decreased self-esteem. Research suggests that almost one of every three rape victims have at least one period of MDD during their lives. And for many of these women, the depression can last for a long period of time. Thoughts about suicide are also common. Studies estimate that one in three women who are raped contemplate suicide, and about one in ten rape victims actually attempt suicide.

## Anger

Many victims of sexual assault report struggling with anger after the assault. Although this is a natural reaction to such a violating event, there is some research that suggests that prolonged, intense anger can interfere with the recovery process and further disrupt a woman's life.

## Shame And Guilt

These feelings are common reactions to sexual assault. Some women blame themselves for what happened or feel shameful about being an assault victim. This reaction can be even stronger among women who are assaulted by someone that they know, or who do not receive support from their friends, family, or authorities following the incident. Shame and guilt can also get in the way of a woman's recovery by preventing her from telling others about what happened and getting assistance.

## Social Problems

Social problems can sometimes arise following a sexual assault. A woman can experience problems in her marital relationship or in her friendships. Sometimes an assault survivor will be too anxious or depressed to want to participate in social activities. Many women report difficulty trusting others after the assault, so it can be difficult to develop new relationships. Performance at work and school can also be affected.

## Sexual Problems

Sexual problems can be among the most long-standing problems experienced by women who are the victims of sexual assault. Women can be afraid of and try to avoid any sexual activity. Or, they may experience an overall decrease in sexual interest and desire.

## Alcohol And Drug Use

Substance abuse can sometimes become problematic for women who are the victims of assault. A large-scale study found that compared to non-victims, rape survivors were three to four times more likely to use marijuana, six times more likely to use cocaine, and ten times more likely to use other major drugs. Often, women will report that they use these substances to control other symptoms related to their assault.

## Posttraumatic Stress Disorder (PTSD)

PTSD involves a pattern of symptoms that some individuals develop after experiencing a traumatic event such as sexual assault. Symptoms of PTSD include repeated thoughts of the assault; memories and nightmares; avoidance of thoughts, feelings, and situations related to the assault; negative changes in thought and feelings; and increased arousal (for example difficulty sleeping and concentrating, jumpiness, irritability). One study that examined PTSD symptoms among women who were raped found that almost all (94 out of 100) women experienced these symptoms during the two weeks immediately following the rape. Nine months later, about 30 out of 100 of the women were still reporting this pattern of symptoms. The National Women's Study reported that almost one of every three all rape victims develop PTSD sometime during their lives.

# What Should I Do If I Have Been Sexually Assaulted? Where Can I Go For Help?

If you were sexually assaulted and are experiencing symptoms that are distressing to you, or symptoms that are interfering with your ability to live a full life, we urge you to talk to a healthcare provider or mental health professional. Depending on the type of problems you are having, a number of therapies may be helpful to you.

The treatment you receive will depend on the symptoms you are experiencing and will be tailored to your needs. Some therapies involve talking about and making sense of the assault in order to reduce the memories and pain associated with the assault. Attending therapy may also involve learning skills to cope with the symptoms associated with the assault. Finally, therapy can help survivors restore meaning to their lives.

Unfortunately, sexual assault is fairly common in our society today. Survivors of sexual assault can experience a wide variety of symptoms, but they do not have to suffer in silence. Mental health professionals can offer a number of effective treatments tailored to the individual woman's needs.

# Chapter 9
# Sexual Abuse of Men

## What Is Sexual Assault?

Sexual assault is any type of sexual contact or behavior that occurs without the explicit consent of the recipient. Falling under the definition of sexual assault are sexual activities as forced sexual intercourse, forcible sodomy, child molestation, incest, fondling, and attempted rape.

## Who Are The Perpetrators Of Male Sexual Assault?

- Those who sexually assault men or boys differ in a number of ways from those who assault only females.

- Boys are more likely than girls to be sexually abused by strangers or by authority figures in organizations such as schools, the church, or athletics programs.

- Those who sexually assault males usually choose young men and male adolescents (the average age is 17 years old) as their victims and are more likely to assault many victims, compared to those who sexually assault females.

- Perpetrators often assault young males in isolated areas where help is not readily available. For instance, a perpetrator who assaults males may pick up a teenage hitchhiker on a remote road or find some other way to isolate his intended victim.

About This Chapter: Text under the heading "What Is Sexual Assault?" is excerpted from "Sexual Assault," Department of Justice (DOJ), April 1, 2016; Text beginning with the heading "Who Are The Perpetrators Of Male Sexual Assault?" is excerpted from "Men And Sexual Trauma," U.S. Department of Veterans Affairs (VA), April 18, 2016.

- As is true about those who assault and sexually abuse women and girls, most perpetrators of males are men. Specifically, men are perpetrators in about 86 out of every 100 (or 86 percent) of male victimization cases.

- Despite popular belief that only gay men would sexually assault men or boys, most male perpetrators identify themselves as heterosexuals and often have consensual sexual relationships with women.

# What Are Some Symptoms Related To Sexual Trauma In Boys And Men?

Particularly when the assailant is a woman, the impact of sexual assault upon men may be downplayed by professionals and the public. However, men who have early sexual experiences with adults report problems in various areas at a much higher rate than those who do not.

## Emotional Disorders

Men and boys who have been sexually assaulted are more likely to suffer from posttraumatic stress disorder (PTSD), anxiety disorders, and depression than those who have never been abused sexually.

## Substance Abuse

Men who have been sexually assaulted have a high incidence of alcohol and drug use. For example, the probability for alcohol problems in adulthood is about 80 out of every 100 (or 80 percent) for men who have experienced sexual abuse, as compared to 11 out of every 100 (or 11 percent) for men who have never been sexually abused.

## Risk Taking Behavior

Exposure to sexual trauma can lead to risk-taking behavior during adolescence, such as running away and other delinquent behaviors. Having been sexually assaulted also makes boys more likely to engage in behaviors that put them at risk for contracting human immunodeficiency virus (HIV) (such as having sex without using condoms).

# Help For Men Who Have Been Sexually Assaulted

Men who have been assaulted often feel stigmatized, which can be the most damaging aspect of the assault. It is important for men to discuss the assault with a caring and unbiased support person, whether that person is a friend, clergyman, or clinician. However, it is vital that this person be knowledgeable about sexual assault and men.

A local rape crisis center may be able to refer men to mental health practitioners who are well-informed about the needs of male sexual assault victims.

## Men and Sexual Trauma

At least 1 out of every 10 (or 10%) of men in our country have suffered from trauma as a result of sexual assault. Like women, men who experience sexual assault may suffer from depression, posttraumatic stress disorder (PTSD), and other emotional problems as a result. However, because men and women have different life experiences due to their different gender roles, emotional symptoms following trauma can look different in men than they do in women.

# Chapter 10
# Incest

One of the least discussed issues related to child abuse is incest. The victims of incest often don't want to talk about it, because of the powerful societal taboo attached to the act. According to U.S. Bureau of Justice Statistics (BJS), about 44 percent of sexual-assault victims are under the age of 18. The data also show that many perpetrators are known to the victims, and one-third are members of the victims' own families. And although it is commonly believed that only men initiate incest, in fact women can be the perpetrators of such abuse. But since this takes place at a much lower rate than incest by men, and since so many of such cases are not reported, it often goes unnoticed.

Considering the gravity of the issue, it is vital to understand what incest is and what can be done about it. This chapter aims to define incest, identify the causes of incest, elucidate the reasons behind the difficulty in sharing information about sexual abuse by a family member, and suggest ways to find help and support for the victim.

## Defining Incest

Incest is defined as sexual contact, including intercourse, between close relatives. In most cultures incest is considered immoral, and in virtually all parts of the United States and many other countries it is also illegal. An adult engaging in incest with a child, however, is considered child abuse under the law, and while legislation pertaining to sexual assault varies, incest with a minor is illegal in all U.S. jurisdictions. The trauma experienced by a young victim of incest can be severe, and the incident can have a serious impact upon the life of the survivor.

"Incest," © 2016 Omnigraphics. Reviewed May 2016.

Although incest can take place between consenting adults, when it occurs between adults and children some common forms include:

- incest between a parent and a child

- incest between an older and younger sibling

- incest between another older relative (for example, an uncle or aunt) and a child

## Signs And Symptoms Of Abuse

To identify whether a child has been a victim of incest, both physical and psychological symptoms must be considered. The physical symptoms include vaginal or rectal pain, vaginal discharge, bleeding, painful urination, bed-wetting, and constipation. The psychological signs include self-harm, nightmares, eating disorders, sleep disorders, aggressive behavior, withdrawal from social interactions, posttraumatic stress disorder (PTSD), lack of concentration, poor performance at school, depression, phobias, and precocious sexual behavior.

## Characteristics Of Incest Offenders

Learning to identify offenders is very important in order to protect children from becoming victims of incest. There are certain characteristics, conditions, and behaviors that are often evident in abusive incest situations. Some examples:

- Adolescent perpetrators often seek victims who are quite young. They tend to abuse the victims for a considerably long period of time. And they may behave more violently than adult perpetrators.

- The absence or unavailability of parents may present the opportunity for incest by siblings or other relatives.

- Dominant or abusive siblings often tend to use incest as a way of expressing their power over the other(s).

- Incest is not always between an adult and a child. Studies have revealed that sibling incest is the most prevalent form of incest.

## The Difficulty In Sharing Information On Sexual Abuse With A Family Member

The very thought of sexual abuse can be disturbing, and talking about it can often be very traumatic. It can become even more difficult to share such incidents if the survivor and the perpetrator are part of the same family.

Some struggles that a victim might face while sharing such information with another family member include:

- concern about the abuser's future

- response or reaction by the family towards the incident, perpetrator, and also the survivor

- negligence or downplaying the issue by the family

- being told that such things are normal in most families

- inability of the family to recognize the incest as a type of abuse

- the victim being unaware of available help or difficulty in finding a trustworthy person

- fear of being harassed by the perpetrator

# Helping The Victims Of Incest

Victims of incest may feel hopeless and can thus be hesitant to seek help. If you observe any symptoms of this type of abuse, some ways to help include:

- **Have a Talk.** By talking to a child who has experienced abuse, you can provide them with comfort and try to ease their pain.

- **Show Faith.** When a victim of abuse reveals their traumatic experience, lend a patient ear. Assure them that you are absolutely serious about what they are saying, and let them know that you are on their side. Then seek the assistance of Child Protective Services.

- **Child Protective Services.** Reporting to Child Protective Services is an option whether the victim is a minor or a vulnerable adult (that is, one who is susceptible to harm due to mental illness, age, or other factors). Contacting the Department of Human Services or the police are other options available to help get assistance for the victim.

## References

1. "Incest," Rape, Abuse and Incest National Network (RAINN), July 2, 2015.

2. "Incest: Informational Fact Sheet," U.S. Marshals Service, U.S. Department of Justice (DOJ), October 5, 2012.

3. Willacy, Hayley, Dr. "Incest," Patient, February 21, 2013.

# Chapter 11

# Stalking

## What Is Stalking?

Stalking is a pattern of repeated and unwanted attention, harassment, contact, or any other course of conduct directed at a specific person that would cause a reasonable person to feel fear.

Stalking can include:

- repeated, unwanted, intrusive, and frightening communications from the perpetrator by phone, mail, and/or e-mail

- repeatedly leaving or sending victim unwanted items, presents, or flowers

- following or laying in wait for the victim at places such as home, school, work, or recreation place

- making direct or indirect threats to harm the victim, the victim's children, relatives, friends, or pets

- damaging or threatening to damage the victim's property

- harassing victim through the Internet

- posting information or spreading rumors about the victim on the Internet, in a public place, or by word of mouth

About This Chapter: Text under the heading "What Is Stalking?" is excerpted from "Stalking," U.S. Department of Justice (DOJ), January 6, 2016; Text beginning with the heading "If You Think You Are Being Stalked" is excerpted from "Violence Against Women," Office on Women's Health (OWH), U.S. Department of Health and Human Services (HHS), September 30, 2015; Text under the heading "Fear, Psychological Distress, And Health Impacts Of Stalking" is excerpted from "Intimate Partner Stalking: Fear, Psychological Distress And Health Impacts," National Institute of Justice (NIJ), U.S. Department of Justice (DOJ), April 20, 2012. Reviewed November 2016.

- obtaining personal information about the victim by accessing public records, using Internet search services, hiring private investigators, going through the victim's garbage, following the victim, contacting victim's friends, family work, or neighbors, etc.

# If You Think You Are Being Stalked

If you think you're being stalked, consider these steps:

- File a complaint with the police. Make sure to tell them about all threats.

- If you are in immediate danger, find a safe place to go, like a police station, friend's house, domestic violence shelter, fire station, or public area. If you can't get out of danger, but can get to a phone, call 911.

- Get a restraining order. A restraining order requires the stalker to stay away from you and not contact you. You can learn how to get a restraining order from a domestic violence shelter, the police, or an attorney in your area.

- Write down every incident. Include the time, date, and other important information.

- Keep evidence such as videotapes, voicemail messages, photos of property damage, and letters. Get names of witnesses.

- Contact support systems to help you, including domestic violence and rape crisis hotlines, domestic violence shelters, counseling services, and support groups. Keep these numbers handy in case you need them.

- Tell important people in your life about the stalking problem, including the police, your employer, family, friends, and neighbors.

- Carry a cellphone at all times so you can call for help.

- Consider changing your phone number (though some people leave their number active to collect evidence). You also can ask the phone company about call blocking and other safety features.

- Secure your home with alarms, locks, and motion-sensitive lights.

# Fear, Psychological Distress, And Health Impacts Of Stalking

Partner stalking victims have higher levels of fear and distress, including anxiety, posttraumatic stress disorder and depression symptoms. Several studies indicate that partner stalking independently contributes to victim fear and distress.

- In general, stalking victimization is associated with a range of fears and significant psychological distress. From a study of stalking victims, of which 68 percent were stalked by an ex-partner, 78 percent had mean scale scores for somatic symptoms, anxiety, social dysfunction and severe depression that were similar to symptoms reported by psychiatric outpatient populations.

- When partner stalking occurs within the context of a current or former relationship that was violent, victim fear and distress is significantly increased.

  - Partner stalking victims with histories of partner violence experienced over three times as many anxiety symptoms as stalking victims with no history of partner violence with the stalker.

  - From a sample of 187 women stalked by an ex-partner, women who experienced violence during the relationship had higher distress levels than women who had not experienced violence during the relationship.

- Studies also suggest that partner stalking contributes uniquely to fear and/or distress after controlling for other forms of partner violence.

  - In a comparison of the experiences of three groups of partner violence victims who had obtained civil protective orders (1) partner violence victims who experienced no stalking and no protective order violations, (2) partner stalking victims who experienced ongoing protective order violations but no stalking, and (3) partner violence victims who experienced protective order violations and stalking, results indicate that stalking victims experience significantly higher fear of future harm and distress than even those with ongoing violations but no stalking.

  - Partner violence victims experience a wide range of fears. A study found that partner stalking victims had significantly higher levels of fear across a variety of dimensions, including physical and sexual assault, ongoing harassment and threats, ongoing coercive control, harm and harassment of friends and family, child threat and interference, economic harm, and public humiliation.

- Partner stalking is associated with sleep and health problems. Health problems may develop from or be exacerbated by the stress and distress from stalking, the cumulative stress and trauma from past violence and abuse and ongoing stalking.

- There is evidence of a dose response relationship with the intensity, frequency, and/or duration of stalking associated with increased fear and distress.

- Several other studies suggest that explicit threats are significantly associated with violence from the partner stalker.

- In one study, researchers concluded, "Though perhaps counter to expectations, it appears that the sense of looming vulnerability that accompanies threats may be more productive of psychological distress in stalking victims than the reality of actual physical assault, which importantly, may precipitate a more sympathetic response, particularly from law enforcement."

- This is consistent with others who have concluded that the harm from stalking is often more psychological than physical.

# Chapter 12
# Sexual Harassment

## What Is Sexual Harassment?

Sexual harassment is conduct that:

1. is sexual in nature

2. is unwelcome

3. denies or limits a student's ability to participate in or benefit from a school's education program.

Sexual harassment can take different forms depending on the harasser and the nature of the harassment. The conduct can be carried out by school employees, other students, and non-employee third parties, such as a visiting speaker. Both male and female students can be victims of sexual harassment and the harasser and the victim can be of the same sex.

The conduct can occur in any school program or activity and can take place in school facilities, on a school bus, or at other off campus locations, such as a school-sponsored field trip or a training program at another location. The conduct can be verbal, nonverbal, or physical.

The judgment and common sense of teachers and school administrators are very important elements in determining whether sexual harassment has occurred and in determining an appropriate response, especially when dealing with young children.

About This Chapter: Text beginning with the heading "What Is Sexual Harassment?" is excerpted from "Sexual Harassment: It's Not Academic," U.S. Department of Education (ED), 2008. Reviewed November 2016; Text under the heading "Youth At Work: Sexual Harassment Is Against The Law" is excerpted from "Youth At Work," U.S. Equal Employment Opportunity Commission (EEOC), April 28, 2016.

# What Are Some Examples Of Sexual Conduct?

Examples of sexual conduct include:

- making sexual propositions or pressuring students for sexual favors

- touching of a sexual nature

- writing graffiti of a sexual nature

- displaying or distributing sexually explicit drawings, pictures, or written materials

- performing sexual gestures or touching oneself sexually in front of others

- telling sexual or dirty jokes

- spreading sexual rumors or rating other students as to sexual activity or performance

- circulating or showing e-mails or websites of a sexual nature

# Is All Physical Contact Sexual In Nature?

No. Legitimate nonsexual touching or conduct generally will not be considered sexual harassment. However, it may rise to that level if it takes on sexual connotations.

# What If The Sexual Conduct Is Criminal In Nature?

Sexual harassment includes conduct that is criminal in nature, such as rape, sexual assault, dating violence, and sexually motivated stalking. Even if a school reports possible criminal conduct to the police, that does not relieve the school of its responsibilities under Title IX.

## Title IX And Sex Discrimination

The U.S. Department of Education's Office for Civil Rights (OCR) enforces, among other statutes, Title IX of the Education Amendments of 1972. Title IX protects people from discrimination based on sex in education programs or activities that receive Federal financial assistance. Title IX states that:

No person in the United States shall, on the basis of sex, be excluded from participation in, be denied the benefits of, or be subjected to discrimination under any education program or activity receiving Federal financial assistance.

Source: Excerpted from "Title IX and Sex Discrimination," U.S. Department of Education (ED), April 29, 2015.

## Must The Sexual Conduct Be Unwelcome?

Yes. Conduct is considered unwelcome if the student did not request or invite it and considered the conduct to be undesirable or offensive. The age of the student, the nature of the conduct, and other relevant factors affect whether a student was capable of welcoming the sexual conduct. A student's submission to the conduct or failure to complain does not always mean that the conduct was welcome.

## When Does Sexual Conduct "Deny Or Limit A Student's Ability To Participate" In Or Benefit From A School's Education Program?

Two general types of sexual conduct can deny or limit a student's ability to participate in or benefit from a school program. As discussed below, teachers and other school employees can engage in either type of conduct, while students and third parties can engage in only one type.

One form of sexual harassment occurs when a teacher or other school employee conditions an educational decision or benefit on the student's submission to unwelcome sexual conduct. If this occurs, it does not matter whether the student resists and suffers the threatened harm or submits to and avoids the threatened harm.

Sexual harassment also occurs when a teacher, school employee, other student, or third party creates a hostile environment that is sufficiently serious to deny or limit a student's ability to participate in or benefit from the school's program. Whether such a hostile environment has been created depends on the particular circumstances of the incident(s). Relevant considerations include, but are not limited to:

- how much of an adverse effect the conduct had on the studends education

- the type, frequency, or duration of the conduct

- the identity age, and sex of the harasser(s) and the victim(s), and the relationship between them

- the number of individuals who engaged in the harassing conduct and at whom the harassment was directed

- the size of the school, location of the incidents, and context in which they occurred

- whether other incidents occurred at the school involving different students

The conduct does not necessarily have to be repetitive. If sufficiently severe, single or isolated incidents Can create a hostile environment.

# Can Young School Children Engage In Sexual Harassment?

School personnel should consider the age and maturity of students in responding to allegations of sexual harassment. When determining whether a young child has committed sexual harassment, it is important for teachers and school administrators to use good judgment and common sense.

# Are Gay And Lesbian Students Protected From Sexual Harassment?

Title IX prohibits harassing conduct that is of a sexual nature if it is unwelcome and denies or limits a student's ability to participate in or benefit from a school's program, regardless of whether the harassment is aimed at gay or lesbian students or is perpetrated by individuals of the same or opposite sex. Title IX does not address discrimination or other issues related to sexual orientation.

# Youth At Work: Sexual Harassment is Against the Law

Sexual harassment is unwelcome or unwanted sexual conduct that is either very serious or occurs frequently. The harasser may be another employee, a supervisor, the company owner or even a customer. The harasser may be male or female. The sexual conduct can be verbal, physical, in writing or in pictures. Illegal sexual harassment creates a hostile or intimidating work place and interferes with an employee's job performance.

## Keep In Mind

**Be Prepared!** Know your rights and responsibilities as an employee or manager.

**Tell the harasser to stop.** If you don't feel comfortable confronting the harasser or the conduct does not stop, tell your employer.

**Report the harassment to your employer.** If your company has a policy on harassment, it should identify who is responsible for handling complaints of harassment. If you are not comfortable talking to that person or your company does not have a harassment policy, talk to your manager or another manager in the company.

**Keep records** including witness names, telephone numbers and addresses. Document how you were treated as an employee.

**Talk to a parent**, teacher, guidance counselor, or another trusted adult about the harassment.

**Act promptly.** Once your employer knows about the harassment, it has a responsibility to stop the harassment. Also, you may not be the only person being harassed by this individual.

**Contact U.S. Equal Employment Opportunity Commission (EEOC)**. The services are free and you do not need a lawyer to file a charge.

# Chapter 13
# Child Pornography

Child pornography is a form of child sexual exploitation. Federal law defines child pornography as any visual depiction of sexually explicit conduct involving a minor (persons less than 18 years old).

Federal law prohibits the production, distribution, importation, reception, or possession of any image of child pornography. A violation of federal child pornography laws is a serious crime, and convicted offenders face fines severe statutory penalties.

## Child Pornography Today

By the mid-1980's, the trafficking of child pornography within the United States was almost completely eradicated through a series of successful campaigns waged by law enforcement. Producing and reproducing child sexual abuse images was difficult and expensive. Anonymous distribution and receipt was not possible, and it was difficult for pedophiles to find and interact with each other. For these reason, child pornographers became lonely and hunted individuals because the purchasing and trading of such images was extremely risky.

Unfortunately, the child pornography market exploded in the advent of the Internet and advanced digital technology. The Internet provides ground for individuals to create, access, and share child sexual abuse images worldwide at the click of a button. Child pornography images are readily available through virtually every Internet technology including websites, email, instant messaging/ICQ, Internet Relay Chat (IRC), newsgroups, bulletin boards, peer-to-peer networks, and social networking sites. Child pornography offenders can connect on Internet

About This Chapter: This chapter includes text excerpted from "Child Pornography," U.S. Department of Justice (DOJ), June 3, 2015.

forums and networks to share their interests, desires, and experiences abusing children in addition to selling, sharing, and trading images.

Moreover, these online communities have promoted communication between child pornography offenders, both normalizing their interest in children and desensitizing them to the physical and psychological damages inflicted on child victims. Online communities may also attract or promote new individuals to get involved in the sexual exploitation of children.

# Victims Of Child Pornography

It is important to distinguish child pornography from the more conventional understanding of the term pornography. Child pornography is a form of child sexual exploitation, and each image graphically memorializes the sexual abuse of that child. Each child involved in the production of an image is a victim of sexual abuse.

While some child sexual abuse images depict children in great distress and the sexual abuse is self-evident, other images may depict children that appear complacent. However, just because a child appears complacent does not mean that sexual abuse did not occur. In most child pornography cases, the abuse is not a one-time event, but rather ongoing victimization that progresses over months or years. It is common for producers of child pornography to groom victims, or cultivate a relationship with a child and gradually sexualize the contact over time. The grooming process fosters a false sense of trust and authority over a child in order to desensitize or break down a child's resistance to sexual abuse. Therefore, even if a child appears complacent in a particular image, it is important to remember that the abuse may have started years before that image was created.

Furthermore, victims of child pornography suffer not just from the sexual abuse inflicted upon them to produce child pornography, but also from knowing that their images can be traded and viewed by others worldwide. Once an image is on the Internet, it is irretrievable and can continue to circulate forever. The permanent record of a child's sexual abuse can alter his or her live forever. Many victims of child pornography suffer from feelings of helplessness, fear, humiliation, and lack of control given that their images are available for others to view in perpetuity.

Unfortunately, emerging trends reveal an increase in the number of images depicting sadistic and violent child sexual abuse, and an increase in the number of images depicting very young children, including toddlers and infants.

# U.S. Federal Law On Child Pornography

Federal law prohibits the production, distribution, reception, and possession of an image of child pornography using or affecting any means or facility of interstate or foreign commerce. Specifically, Section 2251 makes it illegal to persuade, induce, entice, or coerce a minor to engage in sexually explicit conduct for purposes of producing visual depictions of that conduct. Any individual who attempts or conspires to commit a child pornography offense is also subject to prosecution under federal law.

Federal jurisdiction is implicated if the child pornography offense occurred in interstate or foreign commerce. This includes, for example, using the U.S. Mails or common carriers to transport child pornography across state or international borders. Additionally, federal jurisdiction almost always applies when the Internet is used to commit a child pornography violation. Even if the child pornography image itself did not traveled across state or international borders, federal law may be implicated if the materials, such as the computer used to download the image or the CD Rom used to store the image, originated or previously traveled in interstate or foreign commerce.

Lastly, Section 2260 of Title 18, United States Code, prohibits any persons outside of the United States to knowingly produce, receive, transport, ship, or distribute child pornography with intent to import or transmit the visual depiction into the United States.

Any violation of federal child pornography law is a serious crime, and convicted offenders face severe statutory penalties. For example, a first time offender convicted of producing child pornography face fines and a statutory minimum of 15 years to 30 years maximum in prison. A first time offender convicted of transporting child pornography in interstate or foreign commerce faces fines and a statutory minimum of 5 years to 20 years maximum in prison. Convicted offenders may face harsher penalties if the offender has prior convictions or if the child pornography offense occurred in aggravated situations defined as

1. images are violent, sadistic, or masochistic in nature

2. the minor was sexually abused, or

3. the offender has prior convictions for child sexual exploitation. In these circumstances, a convicted offender may face up to life imprisonment.

# Chapter 14

# Commercial Child Sexual Exploitation: Sexual Activities For Money

## Sex Trafficking

Commercial sexual exploitation manifests in numerous forms, such as brothels, sex trafficking, mail order brides, sex tourism, pornography, prostitution, stripping, lap dancing, and phone sex companies. The most common forms of child commercial sexual exploitation are sex trafficking, child pornography, and child sex tourism. One source estimates a child sex trafficker can make as much as $650,000 annually exploiting four children. Exact estimates of prevalence and monetary gain, however, vary extensively because true numbers and figures remain unknown due to a lack of awareness about the issue, general underreporting of the crime, and the difficulties associated with identifying victims and perpetrators.

Sex trafficking is a form of human trafficking, also known as trafficking in persons or modern day slavery. Human trafficking can appear in several other forms, including forced labor, bonded labor, involuntary domestic servitude, child soldier recruitment, and debt bondage among migrant laborers. Recent estimates by global organizations suggest that around 27 million people worldwide are current victims of human trafficking. Sex trafficking is most common in Europe, Central Asia, and the Americas.

Governmental and non-governmental organizations define human trafficking as the exploitation of another person through the use of fraud, coercion, or force. The U.S. Trafficking

About This Chapter: This chapter includes text excerpted from "Commercial Sexual Exploitation Of Children/Sex Trafficking," Office of Juvenile Justice and Delinquency Prevention (OJJDP), U.S. Department of Justice (DOJ), June 3, 2015.

Victims Protection Act of 2000 (TVPA) states that "any commercial sex act if the person is under 18 years of age, regardless of whether any form of coercion is involved, is defined as human trafficking." Therefore, if the victim is considered a minor, then force, fraud, or coercion do not need to be established; the sex act is automatically sex trafficking.

# Characteristics Of Commercial Sexual Exploitation Of Children (CSEC) And Sex Trafficked Children

Identifying victims of CSEC and sex trafficking, can be difficult because of a general lack of public awareness about the issue; the reluctance of many exploited children to identify themselves as victims; and extreme measures taken by exploiters to hide their victims and their crimes. On average, children first fall victim to CSEC between ages 12 and 14. Many youth Child Support Enforcement (CSE) victims tend to come from vulnerable populations with a serious history of previous abuse. Some research suggests victims are now increasingly younger because exploiters are worried about contracting human immunodeficiency virus (HIV) or acquired immunodeficiency syndrome (AIDS) from victims.

> Research on people who are trafficked shows that victims come from all backgrounds, sexes, nations, and economic levels. In a report by the Bureau of Justice Statistics (BJS) on the characteristics of suspected human trafficking incidents, almost 95 percent of sex trafficked victims were female. Over half (54 percent) were 17 years of age or younger.

The degree of traumatization experienced by CSEC victims is well documented. Sexually exploited persons suffer from high rates of:

- posttraumatic stress disorder (PTSD)
- Stockholm syndrome
- memory loss
- aggression and anger issues
- depression
- fear and anxiety
- hostility
- sexually transmitted disease/infection (STD/STI)

- physical trauma from beatings

- emotional and psychological trauma from engaging in unwanted sex

Many risk factors at the societal, community, relationship, and individual levels increase youths' vulnerability to CSEC. The individual level factors include sexual or physical abuse or maltreatment, being a runaway or homeless, system-involvement, such as with the juvenile justice and child welfare systems, being lesbian, gay, bisexual, or transgender, substance abuse, earlier pubertal maturation, and early adversity experiences. In addition, CSEC victims also tend to suffer higher rates of poverty, live in high-crime neighborhoods/environments, have increased rates of mental health issues and higher rates of substance abuse/use or parents who abuse/use substances, and are less likely to be educated or exposed to employment opportunities. Societal risk factors include glorification of pimp culture, objectification of women and girls, gender bias, and widespread use of Internet and social media. Environmental risk factors that allow for higher rates of CSEC and sex trafficking of children include geographical areas with large and international airports, large transient male populations, community violence, street-involved culture/economy, and higher rates of prostitution.

Although research has indicated that most CSEC victims tend to be girls, in recent years the literature has expanded to recognize the victimization of men and boys. It is known that many CSE boys are homeless or runaways and are significantly less likely than girls to have a pimp or other adult exploiting them. Boys and young males likely share many of the risk factors for involvement in CSE as girls, such as child maltreatment and family violence.

# Pathways To Commercial Sexual Exploitation Of Children

CSEC creates a culture that perceives children as commodities that can be bought and sold with little regard for their well-being. In many cases of CSEC and child sex trafficking, victims are exploited through more than one form of abuse. For example, predators may take pornographic images of children, sell those images to other child sex abusers, or use the pictures to advertise the victim for sexual services.

Several core factors often fuel this phenomenon:

- pre-existing adult prostitution markets in communities with high concentrations of street youth

- prior history of child sexual abuse and child sexual assault

- poverty

- large numbers of unattached and transient males in communities, including military personnel, truckers, conventioneers, and sex tourists

- promotion of juvenile prostitution by parents, older siblings, and boyfriends

- recruitment of children by organized crime units for prostitution; and increasingly

- illegal trafficking of children for sexual purposes to the United States from developing countries in Asia, Africa, Central and South America, and Central and Eastern Europe

"Survival sex" is another type of entry into commercial sexual exploitation, where sex is exchanged for necessities such as food or housing. Gang involvement is another common entry for girls into sexual exploitation. Girls are seen as having little to no value other than how they can be used, such as for the sexual gratification of male gang members.

Pimps play another large role in the recruitment and subsequent sexual exploitation of children. They prey upon children from disadvantaged homes/settings and exploit victims through promises of love, food, money, or shelter.

Victims are often unaware where to report their abuse, or they may be so traumatized that they cannot vocalize their experiences. Victims are usually told that their families will be hurt if they report the abuse, so many stay quiet out of fear for their loved ones' safety. Additionally, victims may come from cultures and/or countries where there is a general mistrust or fear of the police or where police and criminal justice corruption are rampant. All these factors likely influence the reporting of abuse and the identification of victims and those responsible for trafficking.

## Treatment Programs For Victims

Victims of trafficking and CSEC often have serious and complicated mental health needs caused by their traumatic experiences. Often victims experience psychological issues such as posttraumatic stress disorder (PTSD). A U.S. Department of Health and Human Services (HHS) report on evidence-based mental health treatment for victims of human trafficking found that some of the "most common presentations for victims of child sexual exploitation are substance-related disorders, dissociative disorders, impulse control, conduct disorder, attention deficit/hyperactivity disorder, antisocial personality traits, and most or all of the Axis IV psychological and environment problems."

Unfortunately, information is lacking about effective methods to treat youth because the identification of PTSD in children has only been recognized more recently compared with adults. The Trauma-Focused Cognitive Behavioral Therapy (TF–CBT) program is one that has been shown to positively impact children who have experienced negative traumatic life events. The TF–CBT treatment intervention is designed to support children ages 3–18 and their parents in overcoming the negative effects of physical and/or sexual abuse. It targets serious emotional problems, including PTSD, stress, anxiety, fear, and depression, by teaching children new skills to process thoughts and emotions that result from the traumatic events. TF–CBT integrates cognitive and behavioral interventions with traditional child-abuse therapies. Its focus is to help children talk directly about their traumatic experiences in a supportive environment.

# Chapter 15

# Use Of Computers In The Sexual Exploitation Of Children

## Types Of Online Child Sexual Exploitation

The Crimes Against Children Research Center (CCRC) delineated three categories of Internet sex crimes against minors. These are:

- **Internet child pornography.** This category included possession/distribution/trade of child pornography and excluded crimes where child pornography was produced. In their nationwide survey of law enforcement, this category was 36 percent of the arrests. Most offenders had images depicting graphic sexual activity with children including penetration of the victim; oral sex; and violence such as bondage, rape, or torture.

- **Internet crimes against identified victims.** This category included online enticement of children, the sending of unwanted sexual materials, and included the production of child pornography. This category encompassed 39 percent of all arrests. The researchers further determined that 20 percent of the arrests were Internet-initiated (the offender had no prior acquaintance with the victim) and in 19 percent of the arrests the offender was a family member or prior acquaintance of the victim who used the Internet to communicate with the victim.

- **Internet solicitations to undercover law enforcement.** This category accounted for 25 percent of the arrests. Approximately one in seven youth ages 10 to 17 who use the Internet receive a sexual solicitation or approach online. Researchers stress that these solicitations were not necessarily from "online predators." Many solicitations could come

About This Chapter: This chapter includes text excerpted from "Preventing Sexual Exploitation Via Internet And Technology," Administration for Children and Families (ACF), U.S. Department of Health and Human Services (HHS), 2010. Reviewed November 2016.

from other youth and when youth knew the sender, and about half of the solicitations were from other youth. Many of the solicitations were brief, rude or vulgar comments or instant messages. Many of the recipients did not view the solicitations as serious or threatening. Four percent of the solicitations (1 in 25) were aggressive solicitations that included attempts to contact the youth offline.

# Which Youth Are Most At Risk?

## Youth At Risk For Online Solicitation

According to research from the CCRC, some teens are at higher risk than others for online sexual exploitation. Those with prior histories of sexual abuse, with sexual orientation concerns, and those with patterns of online or offline risk-taking were at higher risk. Display of sexual content online increases a teen's chances of online victimization. Teens who send personal information or talk online to strangers about sex are at the greatest risk for sexual victimization, since they are the most likely to receive solicitations.

The reality of adolescent sexual development is growing curiosity, knowledge, and experience as youths make the transition from childhood to adulthood. In the past, romances occurred under the scrutiny of parents and peers and others in the social network of the youth. The relative isolation of online relationships may lead to greater intensity and greater disclosure than typically occurs in face-to-face contacts. Adding the factor of youth who lack mature judgment and those who lack emotional regulation skills, then vulnerability is increased.

Posting personal information by itself did not appear to be a particularly risky behavior. Despite admonitions against doing so, it was found that most youth post personal information online. Names, the name of their school, telephone numbers, and general pictures of themselves did not appear to predict risk for online solicitation. Likewise, youth who participated in social networking sites did not appear at increased risk for victimization by online sexual predators. Many youth reported interacting with unknown people on the Internet without receiving unwanted solicitations. Even for youth who were actively seeking to meet new people, the contacts were not likely to be uncomfortable or frightening. Rather, youth who interact in specific ways (talking about sex or sending personal information to unknown persons) were at increased risk. Note that the majority of youth refrain from these risky behaviors. According to the authors, youth who visit chat rooms were likely to have problems with their parents, and to suffer from sadness, loneliness, or depression. These youth with poor social skills may be interacting in chat rooms in order to compensate for problems forming friendships in more conventional ways. The authors comment that online molesters do not appear to be stalking unsuspecting victims but rather seek youth who are vulnerable and susceptible to seduction.

Researchers identified online behaviors that were considered risky. These included:

- interacting online with unknown people

- having unknown people on a buddy list

- talking online to unknown people about sex

- seeking pornography online

- being rude or nasty online

# Law Enforcement Response

Cases involving Internet sex crimes against minors are complex and time-consuming. Many are multijurisdictional and involve more than one law enforcement agency. Many involve collaboration between local and federal law enforcement. They require collaboration and training on how to conduct joint investigations. In spite of difficulties, the rates of dismissal and acquittal are lower than in other types of sex crimes. Internet features such as transcripts of conversations and the actual images sent online may aid in conviction rates and offset the complexity of the prosecution. For that reason, researchers suggest that law enforcement officers should ask all child sexual abuse victims about the ways that the offender talked with them and about everything the offender showed them (including through the Internet), as officers may find evidence such as e-mail correspondence and pictures that might strengthen cases and result in additional charges for crimes such as child pornography. Given that physical evidence is rare in child sexual assault cases, the potential of online evidence should not be ignored.

# Chapter 16

# Sextortion

Sextortion is a type of online sexual exploitation in which individuals coerce victims into providing sexually explicit images or videos of themselves, often in compliance with offenders' threats to post the images publicly or send the images to victims' friends and family. The Federal Bureau of Investigation (FBI) has seen a significant increase in sextortion activity against children who use the Internet, typically ages 10 to 17, but any age child can become a victim of sextortion.

## Technical Details

The FBI is seeking to warn parents, educators, caregivers, and children about the dangers of sextortion. Sending just one inappropriate image to another person online could become the catalyst for sextortion if that image, shared publicly or with their family and friends, is considered compromising to the victim. Offenders easily misrepresent themselves online to appear to be friendly and age appropriate or simply an adult who will listen to a child. This relationship can be manipulated to groom the child to eventually send inappropriate images or video to the offender. Furthermore, children may send images or videos to a known individual on purpose, but an offender may come into possession of those images or videos through the sextortion of the original recipient or if the original recipient puts the image on the Internet and the offender comes across it. Younger children can become victims when their friend or sibling is being sextorted and the offender threatens to make images or videos public if their requests to include the sexual abuse of younger children in the images or videos are not satisfied.

---

About This Chapter: This chapter includes text excerpted from "Sextortion Affecting Thousands Of U.S. Children," Federal Bureau of Investigation (FBI), June 20, 2016.

# Threat

Children tend to be trusting online and will befriend people of any age or sex they may not know. Offenders take advantage of this naivety and target children who openly engage others online or have a strong social networking presence. In most instances, they openly post pictures or videos of themselves. Offenders can gain information from the online presence of potential victims by reviewing posts and "friends lists" and pose as an acquaintance, another teen from the same or a different school, or a stranger with similar interests. "Friends lists" may serve as a source to identify additional victims once the sextortion process starts. Once a child becomes a victim of sextortion, the victimization may last for years. Victims have reported having to meet demands for sexually explicit images and videos multiple times per day. The FBI has identified cases in which children committed suicide, attempted suicide, or engaged in other acts of self–harm due to their sextortion victimization. In one instance, the victim purposely engaged in activity that put them in the hospital to get a break from their offender's demands. As soon as the victim was released from the hospital, the victimization continued.

# Defense

Sextortion is a crime. The coercion of a child by an adult to produce what is considered child pornography carries heavy penalties, which can include up to life sentences for the offender. The FBI does not treat a child as an offender in the production of child pornography as a result of their sextortion or coercion. In order for the victimization to stop, children typically have to come forward to someone—normally a parent, teacher, caregiver, or law enforcement. The embarrassment of the activity a child was forced to engage in is what typically prevents them from coming forward. Sextortion offenders may have hundreds of victims around the world, so coming forward to help law enforcement identify the offender may prevent countless other incidents of sexual exploitation to that victim and others.

The following measures may help educate and prevent children from becoming victims of this type of sexual exploitation:

- Make children aware that anything done online may be available to others;

- Make sure children's apps and social networking sites' privacy settings are set to the strictest level possible;

- Anyone who asks a child to engage in sexually explicit activity online should be reported to a parent, guardian, or law enforcement;

- It is not a crime for a child to send sexually explicit images to someone if they are compelled to do so, so victims should not be afraid to tell law enforcement if they are being sexually exploited;

- Parents should put personal computers in a central location in the home;

- Parents should review and approve apps downloaded to smart phones and mobile devices and monitor activity on those devices;

- Ensure an adult is present and engaged when children communicate via webcam; and

- Discuss Internet safety with children before they engage in any online activity and maintain those discussions as children become teenagers.

What to do if you believe you are or someone you know is the victim of sextortion:

- Contact your local law enforcement agency, your local FBI field office, or the National Center for Missing and Exploited Children at 1-800-THE-LOST (1-800-843-5678) or Cybertipline.org;

- Do not delete anything before law enforcement is able to review it; and

- Tell law enforcement everything about the encounters you had online—it may be embarrassing, but it is necessary to find the offender.

# Part Two
## Violence And The Teen Experience

# Chapter 17

# Risk Factors For Youth Violence: An Overview

## Risk Factors For The Perpetration Of Youth Violence

Research on youth violence has increased our understanding of factors that make some populations more vulnerable to victimization and perpetration. Risk factors increase the likelihood that a young person will become violent. However, risk factors are not direct causes of youth violence; instead, risk factors contribute to youth violence.

> **What Is A Risk Factor?**
>
> A risk factor is a characteristic that increases the likelihood of a person becoming a victim or perpetrator of violence.
>
> Source: "Preventing Youth Violence: Opportunities For Action," Centers for Disease Control and Prevention (CDC), June 2014.

Research associates the following risk factors with perpetration of youth violence:

### Individual Risk Factors

- History of violent victimization

- Attention deficits, hyperactivity or learning disorders

---

About This Chapter: This chapter includes text excerpted from "Youth Violence: Risk And Protective Factors," Centers for Disease Control and Prevention (CDC), March 21, 2016.

- History of early aggressive behavior
- Involvement with drugs, alcohol or tobacco
- Low IQ
- Poor behavioral control
- Deficits in social cognitive or information-processing abilities
- High emotional distress
- History of treatment for emotional problems
- Antisocial beliefs and attitudes
- Exposure to violence and conflict in the family

## Family Risk Factors

- Authoritarian childrearing attitudes
- Harsh, lax or inconsistent disciplinary practices
- Low parental involvement
- Low emotional attachment to parents or caregivers
- Low parental education and income
- Parental substance abuse or criminality
- Poor family functioning
- Poor monitoring and supervision of children

## Peer And Social Risk Factors

- Association with delinquent peers
- Involvement in gangs
- Social rejection by peers
- Lack of involvement in conventional activities
- Poor academic performance
- Low commitment to school and school failure

## Community Risk Factors

- Diminished economic opportunities

- High concentrations of poor residents

- High level of transiency

- High level of family disruption

- Low levels of community participation

- Socially disorganized neighborhoods

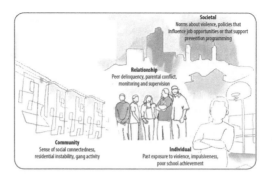

*Figure 17.1.* Risk Factors For Youth Violence

# Protective Factors For The Perpetration Of Youth Violence

Protective factors buffer young people from the risks of becoming violent. These factors exist at various levels. To date, protective factors have not been studied as extensively or rigorously as risk factors. However, identifying and understanding protective factors are equally as important as researching risk factors.

## What Is A Protective Factor?

A protective factor is a characteristic that decreases the likelihood of a person becoming a victim or perpetrator of violence or buffers against the effects of risk factors.

*Source: "Preventing Youth Violence: Opportunities For Action," Centers for Disease Control and Prevention (CDC), June 2014.*

Most research is preliminary. Studies propose the following protective factors:

## Individual Protective Factors

- Intolerant attitude toward deviance
- High IQ
- High grade point average (as an indicator of high academic achievement)
- Positive social orientation
- Highly developed social skills/competencies
- Highly developed skills for realistic planning
- Religiosity

## Family Protective Factors

- Connectedness to family or adults outside the family
- Ability to discuss problems with parents
- Perceived parental expectations about school performance are high
- Frequent shared activities with parents
- Consistent presence of parent during at least one of the following: when awakening, when arriving home from school, at evening mealtime or going to bed
- Involvement in social activities
- Parental / family use of constructive strategies for coping with problems (provision of models of constructive coping)

## Peer And Social Protective Factors

- Possession of affective relationships with those at school that are strong, close, and pro-socially oriented
- Commitment to school (an investment in school and in doing well at school)
- Close relationships with non-deviant peers
- Membership in peer groups that do not condone antisocial behavior
- Involvement in prosocial activities

- Exposure to school climates that characterized by:

  - Intensive supervision

  - Clear behavior rules

  - Consistent negative reinforcement of aggression

  - Engagement of parents and teachers

# Chapter 18

# Oppositional Defiant Disorder And Conduct Disorder

Children sometimes argue, are aggressive, or act angry or defiant around adults. A behavior disorder may be diagnosed when these disruptive behaviors are uncommon for the child's age at the time, persist over time, or are severe. Because behavior disorders involve acting out and showing unwanted behavior towards others they are often called externalizing disorders.

## Oppositional Defiant Disorder

When children act out persistently so that it causes serious problems at home, in school, or with peers, they may be diagnosed with oppositional defiant disorder (ODD). ODD usually starts before 8 years of age, but no later than by about 12 years of age. Children with ODD are more likely to act oppositional or defiant around people they know well, such as family members, a regular care provider, or a teacher. Children with ODD show these behaviors more often than other children their age.

Examples of ODD behaviors include:

- Often being angry or losing one's temper

- Often arguing with adults or refusing to comply with adults' rules or requests

- Often resentful or spiteful

- Deliberately annoying others or becoming annoyed with others

- Often blaming other people for one's own mistakes or misbehavior

---

About This Chapter: This chapter includes text excerpted from "Children's Mental Health," Centers for Disease Control and Prevention (CDC), April 22, 2016.

# Conduct Disorder

Conduct disorder (CD) is diagnosed when children show an ongoing pattern of aggression toward others, and serious violations of rules and social norms at home, in school, and with peers. These rule violations may involve breaking the law and result in arrest. Children with CD are more likely to get injured and may have difficulties getting along with peers.

Examples of CD behaviors include:

- Breaking serious rules, such as running away, staying out at night when told not to, or skipping school

- Being aggressive in a way that causes harm, such as bullying, fighting, or being cruel to animals

- Lying, stealing, or damaging other people's property on purpose

# Treatment For Disruptive Behavior Disorders

Starting treatment early is important. Treatment is most effective if it fits the needs of the specific child and family. The first step to treatment is to talk with a healthcare provider. A comprehensive evaluation by a mental health professional may be needed to get the right diagnosis. Some of the signs of behavior problems, such as not following rules in school, could be related to learning problems which may need additional intervention. For younger children, the treatment with the strongest evidence is behavior therapy training for parents, where a therapist helps the parent learn effective ways to strengthen the parent-child relationship and respond to the child's behavior. For school-age children and teens, an often-used effective treatment is a combination of training and therapy that includes the child, the family, and the school.

# Prevention Of Disruptive Behavior Disorders

It is not known exactly why some children develop disruptive behavior disorders. Many factors may play a role, including biological and social factors. It is known that children are at greater risk when they are exposed to other types of violence and criminal behavior, when they experience maltreatment or harsh or inconsistent parenting, or when their parents have mental health conditions like substance use disorders, depression, or attention-deficit/hyperactivity disorder (ADHD). The quality of early childhood care also can impact whether a child develops behavior problems.

# Chapter 19

# Electronic Aggression

## Technology And Youth Violence

Young people are using media technology, including cell phones, personal data assistants, and the Internet, to communicate with others in the United States and throughout the world. Communication avenues, such as text messaging, chat rooms, and social networking websites, such as Twitter and Facebook, allow youth to easily develop relationships, some with people they have never met in person.

Media technology has many potential benefits for youth. It allows young people to communicate with family and friends on a regular basis. This technology also provides opportunities to make rewarding social connections for those teens and pre-teens who have difficulty developing friendships in traditional social settings or because of limited contact with same-aged peers. In addition, regular Internet access allows young people to quickly increase their knowledge on a wide variety of topics.

However, the explosion in communication tools and avenues does not come without possible risks. Youth can use electronic media to embarrass, harass or threaten their peers. Increasing numbers of teens and pre-teens are becoming victims of this new form of violence. Although many different terms, such as "cyberbullying," "Internet harassment," and "Internet bullying," have been used to describe this type of violence, "electronic aggression" is the term that most accurately captures all types of violence that occur electronically. Like traditional forms of youth violence, electronic aggression is associated with emotional distress and

About This Chapter: Text under the heading "Technology And Youth Violence" is excerpted from "Electronic Aggression," Centers for Disease Control and Prevention (CDC), September 22, 2016; Text under the heading "Sources For Electronic Aggression" is excerpted from "Violent Content Research Act Of 2013," Library of Congress (LOC), U.S. House of Representatives, December 17, 2013. Reviewed November 2016.

conduct problems at school. In fact, recent research suggests that youth who are victimized electronically are also very likely to also be victimized off-line. That is, they are likely to be sexually harassed, psychologically or emotionally abused by a caregiver, witness an assault with a weapon, and raped.

# Sources For Electronic Aggression

There is a broad field of research examining the impact of violent media content on aggression in children and adolescents. The American Academy of Pediatrics (AAP) has stated that media violence is a public health issue. The AAP's policy statement on the issue begins as follows: "Exposure to violence in media, including television, movies, music, and video games, represents a significant risk to the health of children and adolescents." In reaching this conclusion, the AAP cites American and cross-cultural studies, field experiments, cross-sectional studies, and longitudinal studies involving children, teens, and young adults.

Federal agencies also have reached a similar conclusion. In a 2007 report on violent television programming and its impact on children, the Federal Communications Commission (FCC) agreed with the views of the then Surgeon General that there was "strong evidence that exposure to violence in the media can increase aggressive behavior in children, at least in the short term." The FCC went on to detail the state of the research at that time on the effects of violent video programming, noting that "a significant number of health professionals, parents, and members of the general public are concerned about television violence and its effect on children."

In 2012, a special commission appointed by the International Society for Research on Aggression released its findings about the state of the research into the impacts of media violence. The report found that "exposure to violent media can increase not only aggressive behavior in a variety of forms, but also aggressive thoughts, aggressive feelings, psychological arousal, and decrease prosocial behavior" and further found that the "effects are remarkably consistent regardless of the type of medium, age, gender, or where the person lives in the world."

Despite the findings in these reports, there is not universal agreement on the impacts of such media violence on children. In 2011, the Supreme Court overturned a California law banning the sales of certain violent video games to minors. A key element of that decision was the finding by the majority of the Court that scientific literature demonstrating the ill-effects of video game and media violence on children was not persuasive. While studies may suggest a correlation between violent video games and aggressive behavior, the majority of the Court argued that causation had not been demonstrated. In addition, the Court's majority contended that the effects on children from video violence are small and indistinguishable from the effects of other media that enjoy full First Amendment protection (e.g., aggression resulting from reading Lord of the Flies, The Odyssey, or even comic books.) Some research has backed up these arguments with findings that either the impact of violent media is dwarfed by other factors—such as family violence—or that any impacts media violence may have on short-term aggression do not translate into real-world violence.

For instance, in 2008, researchers conducted two studies examining the relationship between exposure to violent video games and aggression and found "no link, either causal or correlational between violent-video-game playing and aggressive or violent acts." The lead researcher on that 2008 study, Christopher Ferguson of Texas A&M University, has also raised questions concerning the validity of other research exploring possible links between exposure to media violence and aggression. His 2009 meta-analytic review of existing studies on the impact of violent media on aggressive behavior found publication bias in this field, and concluded that "the perception of the strength, consistency, and generalizability of existing media violence research may be greatly overstated."

With video game interactivity increasing, and the sources for video programming expanding to online, mobile, and on demand platforms, it is important to have a respected, neutral, expert third party to take a comprehensive look at the state of the research on violent content and its impact on the well-being of children. As proposed in S. 134, the National Academy of Sciences (NAS) independent view on the current state of research and a research plan for future research in this area could inform research by other organizations, including the Centers for Disease Control and Prevention (CDC), and provide guidance to lawmakers.

# Chapter 20
# Teen Drug Use And Violence

It sounds like the name of a new reality show, right? But in *real* real life, there is a connection between people in abusive dating relationships, and drugs and alcohol.

Actually, it's a two-way street. Drugs and alcohol increase the risk for dating violence, and people who are victims of dating violence are at increased risk for using drugs and alcohol.

Being drunk or drugged can make someone more likely to physically or emotionally hurt a person they're in a relationship with. Drugs and alcohol make it harder to keep your emotions in check and to make the right choices. They also make it easier to act impulsively without thinking through the consequences. And the people on the receiving end of that abuse are more likely to turn to drugs and alcohol to cope with the depression and anxiety that result from being victimized.

Abuse between teens in a romantic relationship is known as Teen Dating Violence. It happens when one person intentionally hurts the other—or when they both do it to each other. Dating violence can be emotional, physical, and/or sexual, and it also includes stalking. It can be with a current or former partner. It can happen in person or electronically. And it has real consequences for a person's health, today and in the future.

Abusive relationships don't always start out that way. Often, they start with teasing, or periods of jealously or being controlling. But as with many unhealthy behaviors, over time it can get worse. For nearly 10 percent of high school students surveyed by the Centers for Disease

About This Chapter: Text in this chapter begins with excerpts from "Love And Drugs And Violence," NIDA for Teens, National Institute on Drug Abuse (NIDA), March 26, 2015; Text under the heading "Treating Principles" is excerpted from "Drug Addiction Treatment In The Criminal Justice System," National Institute on Drug Abuse (NIDA), April 2014.

Control and Pervention (CDC) in 2013, "worse" means that in the last year they were hit, slapped, or physically hurt by their partner.

The best way to avoid teen dating violence (for those of you allowed to date!) is by having healthy relationships. This doesn't mean there isn't any conflict in the relationship, because that isn't realistic—even for the most in-love people ever. It means both people learning how to resolve their differences respectfully. That can make all the difference.

There were differences in the types of drugs used before a dating violence incident vs. non-dating violence incidents.

For example, some youth tended to use alcohol alone or in combination with marijuana just before a non-dating violence incident occurred and tended to abuse prescription sedatives (Xanax or Valium) and/or opioids (like Vicodin and OxyContin) before a dating violence incident occurred.

*Source: "Drug Use And Violence: An Unhappy Relationship," NIDA for Teens, National Institute on Drug Abuse (NIDA), March 26, 2015.*

# Treatment Principles

*Principles for Drug Abuse Treatment for Criminal Justice Populations*: A Research-Based Guide provides research-based principles of addiction treatment. The 13 principles are:

1. Drug addiction is a brain disease that affects behavior.

2. Recovery from drug addiction requires effective treatment, followed by management of the problem over time.

3. Treatment must last long enough to produce stable behavioral change.

4. Assessment is the first step in treatment.

5. Tailoring services to fit the needs of the individual is an important part of effective drug use treatment for criminal justice populations.

6. Drug use during treatment should be carefully monitored.

7. Treatment should target factors that are associated with criminal behavior.

8. Criminal justice supervision should incorporate treatment planning for drug using offenders, and treatment providers should be aware of correctional supervision requirements.

9. Continuity of care is essential for drug users re-entering the community.

10. A balance of rewards and sanctions encourages pro-social behavior and treatment participation.

11. Offenders with co-occurring drug use and mental health problems often require an integrated treatment management approach.

12. Medications are an important part of treatment for many drug using offenders.

13. Treatment planning for drug using offenders who are living in or re-entering the community should include strategies to prevent and treat serious, chronic medical conditions, such as HIV/AIDS, hepatitis B and C, and tuberculosis.

# Chapter 21

# The Relationship Between Substance Abuse And Violence Against Women

## Domestic Violence And Substance Abuse

Research indicates a significant correlation between substance abuse and domestic violence victims. The presence of alcohol or other drugs in domestic violence incidents raises important concerns about victims' safety and their capacity to respond to threats or acts of violence. It does *not* mean, however, that the presence of such substances *caused* the abuse to occur. Moreover, substance abuse is sometimes wrongly considered by law enforcement, justice professionals, substance abuse treatment professionals, and batterers intervention professionals to be a *causal*, as opposed to *correlating*, factor in domestic violence within the framework of both the abuser and the victim.

The following facts represent several findings about the correlation between substance abuse and domestic violence:

- Being a victim of domestic violence is associated with an increased incidence of substance abuse.

- Approximately 50 percent of all female alcoholics have been victims of domestic violence.

- In a research study conducted by medical personnel and researchers who accompanied police in Memphis as they responded to nighttime calls for assistance, 42 percent of victims of domestic violence used alcohol or drugs on the day of the assault according to their own reports or reports of family members. Fifteen percent had used cocaine, and about half of those using cocaine said their batterers had forced them to use it.

About This Chapter: This chapter includes text excerpted from "Substance Abuse And Victimization," National Criminal Justice Reference Service (NCJRS), 2000. Reviewed November 2016.

- In a study of murder in families, half of the victims in spouse murders had consumed alcohol before the crime.

- Having a partner who abuses chemicals is more likely to generate substance abuse in women.

- A batterer may also be the victim's drug supplier, which complicates the situation.

- Drug- or alcohol-involved victims of partner abuse may not be taken as seriously by professionals. Substance abuse may be viewed as a reason for the abuse, and this is often an inaccurate assessment.

- Victims of domestic violence are more likely to receive prescriptions for and become dependent on tranquilizers, sedatives, stimulants, and painkillers and are more likely to abuse alcohol.

# Sexual Assault And Substance Abuse

Alcohol and other drugs are often present in both victims and offenders of sexual assault. Similar to crimes of domestic violence, this can wrongly be construed as a *causal* rather than a *correlating* factor to the offense. There is overwhelming evidence that victims of sexual assault and rape are much more likely to use alcohol and other drugs to cope with the trauma of victimization than nonvictims:

- Rape victims were 5.3 times more likely than nonvictims to have used prescription drugs nonmedically.

- Rape victims were 3.4 times more likely to have used marijuana than nonvictims.

- Victims of rape were six times more likely to have used cocaine than their counterparts who were not raped.

- Compared to women who had not been raped, rape victims were 10.1 times more likely to have used "hard drugs" other than cocaine.

- Drinking by the victim, the assailant, or both is involved in over half of sexual assaults.

# Substance Abuse, Adolescents, And Adolescent Victims

Research reveals that adolescents who use and abuse substances are more prone to serious psychological and behavioral problems. Youth who are victimized by physical or sexual abuse are much more likely to develop chemical dependencies:

- In a nationally representative sample, youth who experienced either physical or sexual abuse or assault were twice as likely as their nonvictimized peers to report past-year alcohol or other drug abuse or dependence.

- This same national study found that youth who witnessed violence (including domestic violence and violence among their peers) were three times as likely to experience substance use disorders.

- Among 12-to-17-year-old current drinkers, 31 percent had extreme levels of psychological distress, and 39 percent exhibited serious behavioral problems.

In 1995, the National Crime Victims Research and Treatment Center (NCVC) at the Medical University of South Carolina conducted the first-ever National Study of Adolescents (NSA) that examined victimization, mental health, and substance abuse issues among teenagers. A telephonic survey of 4,023 adolescents ages twelve to seventeen determined that, based on U.S. Census 1995 estimates of the U.S. population of adolescents of 22.3 million: 1.8 million adolescents have been sexually assaulted; 3.9 million have been physically assaulted; 2.1 million have been subjected to physically abusive punishment; and 8.8 million have witnessed violence. Significantly, over one half of adolescent victims said that their first use of substances occurred after the year they were first assaulted (53.8 percent for alcohol, 47.8 percent for marijuana, and 63.5 percent for hard drugs).

Much of the knowledge gained from the NSA raises crucial issues that cross over lines of research, policy, and practice. As such, collaborative efforts to address these concerns should be encouraged among professionals in the fields of victim assistance, criminal and juvenile justice, mental health, and substance abuse. Among the many NSA recommendations for public policymakers are three that are specific to youth victimization and substance abuse:

1. The NSA found that many violence victims had comorbid posttraumatic stress disorer (PTSD) and substance use/abuse/dependence problems, and that victimization is an important pathway to substance abuse and delinquency. These findings imply that effective mental health treatment for adolescent victims is important not only to relieve postvictimization mental health problems, but also to prevent future substance use and delinquent or criminal behavior. Therefore, mechanisms should be developed to ensure that funding is available to provide mental health counseling to adolescent victims who need it, irrespective of their ability to pay or whether they qualify for crime victim compensation.

2. Policies should promote the primary and secondary prevention of child victimization as part of a comprehensive plan for preventing youth substance use and delinquency.

Effective and efficient prevention begins as early as possible in the risk factor chain. Results of this study suggest that victimization and its effects are strong and primary correlates with youth substance abuse and delinquency, even when controlling for other risk factors. Therefore, prevention of these early primary experiences will contribute to preventing these secondary problems.

3. Policies should encourage early identification of and intervention with victimized children (secondary and tertiary prevention). All child victimizations cannot be prevented. However, if more can be recognized and effective interventions provided to child victims, it is likely that at least some of the long-term negative effects leading to substance use and delinquency can be mitigated. Therefore, policies should encourage proactive—rather than reactive—approaches to identifying victimized youth, and should promote effective and rapid intervention for victimization-related problems that are related to the development of substance use and delinquency.

The NSA's emphasis on collaborative initiatives to respond to substance use and abuse among adolescent victims extended to practitioners as well, with three important recommendations:

1. Mental health professionals who work with children and adolescents should be informed about the high rates of victimization that occur among children and adolescents, and about the extent to which victimization serves as a risk factor for PTSD, substance use/abuse/dependence, and delinquency. In addition, they should be encouraged to screen for victimization experiences among child and adolescent clients. Substance abuse treatment programs for adolescents should do likewise.

2. Victim assistance professionals in the criminal and juvenile justice systems should establish relationships with mental health professionals who are knowledgeable about crime victims' mental health issues. Criminal and juvenile justice practitioners and victim service providers should establish or enhance professional relationships with substance abuse professionals in order to effectively address issues of substance use, abuse, and dependency among adolescents and children who have been victimized.

3. Mental health programs dealing with child victims should incorporate substance abuse and delinquency prevention components into their protocols. While mental health programs designed to reduce common psychological problems associated with child victimization are common, few include specific interventions for reducing substance use onset, substance abuse, or conduct and delinquency problems. Given the findings of the NSA, mental health programs should incorporate these prevention components as a regular part of their victimization treatment protocols.

# Chapter 22
# Teen Dating Violence

Dating violence is a type of intimate partner violence. It occurs between two people in a close relationship. The nature of dating violence can be physical, emotional, or sexual.

- **Physical**—This occurs when a partner is pinched, hit, shoved, slapped, punched, or kicked.

- **Psychological/Emotional**—This means threatening a partner or harming his or her sense of self-worth. Examples include name calling, shaming, bullying, embarrassing on purpose, or keeping him/her away from friends and family.

- **Sexual**—This is forcing a partner to engage in a sex act when he or she does not or cannot consent. This can be physical or nonphysical, like threatening to spread rumors if a partner refuses to have sex.

- **Stalking**—This refers to a pattern of harassing or threatening tactics that are unwanted and cause fear in the victim.

Dating violence can take place in person or electronically, such as repeated texting or posting sexual pictures of a partner online.

Unhealthy relationships can start early and last a lifetime. Teens often think some behaviors, like teasing and name calling, are a "normal" part of a relationship. However, these behaviors can become abusive and develop into more serious forms of violence.

About This Chapter: Text in this chapter begins with excerpts from "Understanding Teen Dating Violence," Centers for Disease Control and Prevention (CDC), May 20, 2016; Text under the heading "What Are The Consequences Of Dating Violence" is excerpted from "Teen Dating Violence," Centers for Disease Control and Prevention (CDC), July 21, 2016.

## Why Is Dating Violence A Public Health Problem?

Dating violence is a widespread issue that has serious long-term and short-term effects. Many teens do not report it because they are afraid to tell friends and family.

- Among high school students who dated, 21 percent of females and 10 percent of males experienced physical and/ or sexual dating violence.

- Among adult victims of rape, physical violence, and/or stalking by an intimate partner, 22 percent of women and 15 percent of men first experienced some form of partner violence between 11 and 17 years of age.

## How Does Dating Violence Affect Health?

Dating violence can have a negative effect on health throughout life. Youth who are victims are more likely to experience symptoms of depression and anxiety, engage in unhealthy behaviors, like using tobacco, drugs, and alcohol, or exhibit antisocial behaviors and think about suicide. Youth who are victims of dating violence in high school are at higher risk for victimization during college.

## Who Is At Risk For Dating Violence?

Factors that increase risk for harming a dating partner include the following:

- Belief that dating violence is acceptable

- Depression, anxiety, and other trauma symptoms

- Aggression towards peers and other aggressive behavior

- Substance use

- Early sexual activity and having multiple sexual partners

- Having a friend involved in dating violence

- Conflict with partner

- Witnessing or experiencing violence in the home

## How Can We Prevent Dating Violence?

The ultimate goal is to stop dating violence before it starts. Strategies that promote healthy relationships are vital. During the preteen and teen years, young people are learning skills they need to form positive relationships with others. This is an ideal time to promote healthy relationships and prevent patterns of dating violence that can last into adulthood. Many prevention strategies are proven to prevent or reduce dating violence. Some effective school-based programs change norms, improve problem-solving, and address dating violence in addition to other youth risk behaviors, such as substance use and sexual risk behaviors. Other programs prevent dating violence through changes to the school environment or training influential adults, like parents/caregivers and coaches, to work with youth to prevent dating violence.

An evaluation of the *Coaching Boys Into Men* program showed that high school male athlete participants increased intentions and positive behavior to intervene on peers' dating and sexual violence behaviors relative to control athletes. At the one-year follow-up, the perpetration of dating violence was also less among program participants.

*Source: "Drug Use And Violence: An Unhappy Relationship," NIDA for Teens, National Institute on Drug Abuse (NIDA), March 26, 2015.*

# What Are The Consequences Of Dating Violence?

As teens develop emotionally, they are heavily influenced by experiences in their relationships. Healthy relationship behaviors can have a positive effect on a teen's emotional development. Unhealthy, abusive, or violent relationships can have severe consequences and short- and long-term negative effects on a developing teen. Youth who experience dating violence are more likely to experience the following:

- Symptoms of depression and anxiety

- Engagement in unhealthy behaviors, such as tobacco and drug use, and alcohol

- Involvement in antisocial behaviors

- Thoughts about suicide

- Additionally, youth who are victims of dating violence in high school are at higher risk for victimization during college.

# Chapter 23

# Physical Fighting Among Teenagers

Youth homicide in the United States is a significant public health issue. Homicide is the third leading cause of death among young people aged 10–24 years, responsible for more deaths in this age group than the next seven leading causes of death combined. For each young homicide victim, we lose an entire lifetime of contributions to families, potential employers, and communities. The number of youth who are physically harmed but do not die as the result of youth violence is significantly higher. For every young homicide victim, there were approximately 142 youth with nonfatal physical assault-related injuries treated in U.S. emergency departments. A total of 599,336 youth aged 10–24 years (928 per 100,000) were treated in U.S. emergency departments for nonfatal physical assault-related injuries in 2012. This means that each day approximately 13 young people are victims of homicide and an additional 1,642 are treated in emergency departments for physical assault-related injuries.

Official data from death certificates and emergency departments are critical to helping understand and address youth violence, but they only tell part of the story. The full extent of the violence that youth perpetrate and experience as victims goes far beyond these data sources. The Youth Risk Behavior Survey conducted by Centers for Disease Control and Prevention (CDC) in 2013 indicates that 24.7 percent of high school students reported having been in at least one physical fight in the year before the survey.

About This Chapter: Text in this chapter begins with excerpts from "Preventing Youth Violence: Opportunities For Action," Centers for Disease Control and Prevention (CDC), June 2014; Text under the heading "Violence Against Peers" is excerpted from "Girls Study Group," Office of Juvenile Justice and Delinquency Prevention (OJJDP), U.S. Department of Justice (DOJ), May 2008. Reviewed November 2016; Text under the heading "Physical Fighting In School" is excerpted from "CDC Releases Youth Risk Behaviors Survey Results," Centers for Disease Control and Prevention (CDC), June 9, 2016.

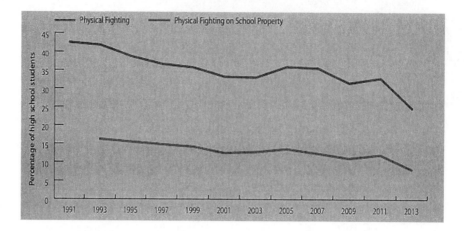

**Figure 23.1.** Prevalence Of Physical Fighting Among High School Students In The United States, 1991–2013

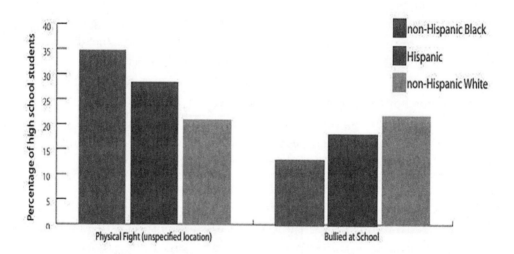

**Figure 23.2.** Physical Fighting And Bullying Among High School Students In The United States By Race/Ethnicity, 2013

# Violence Against Peers

Girls and boys are more likely to attack their same-sex peers than any other type of victim. A study found that, regardless of gender, the most common reasons youth were violent toward peers was to punish them for something done or said, to get them to back down from offensive actions, and in self-defense. Physical touching, often aggressive, was the most frequent immediate precipitator of a violent incident. The second most common trigger of peer violence was negative verbal exchanges. Other researchers have examined the relationship between physical violence and relational aggression, which includes trying to damage the social standing or self-esteem of peers by using verbal rejection, gossip, rumor spreading, and social ostracism.

In some social and cultural groups, the influences against fighting weaken the connection of relational aggression to physical violence; specifically, it was found that among middle-class African American youth, episodes of relational aggression were followed by nonphysical confrontations and ostracism but not by physical fighting.

## What We Know About Girls and Violence

Available evidence based on arrest, victimization, and self-report data suggests that although girls are currently arrested more for simple assaults than previously, the actual incidence of their being seriously violent has not changed much over the last two decades. This suggests that increases in arrests may be attributable more to changes in enforcement policies than to changes in girls' behavior. Juvenile female involvement in violence has not increased relative to juvenile male violence. There is no burgeoning national crisis of increasing serious violence among adolescent girls.

Although more information is needed, current literature suggests that girls' violence occurs in the following situations, for the following reasons:

- **Peer violence.** Girls fight with peers to gain status, to defend their sexual reputation, and in self-defense against sexual harassment.

- **Family violence.** Girls fight more frequently at home with parents than do boys, who engage more frequently in violence outside the household. Girls' violence against parents is multidimensional: for some, it represents striking back against what they view as an overly controlling structure; for others, it is a defense against or an expression of anger stemming from being sexually and or physically abused by members of the household.

- **Violence within schools.** When girls fight in schools, they may do so as a result of teacher labeling, in self-defense, or out of a general sense of hopelessness.

- **Violence within disadvantaged neighborhoods.** Girls in disadvantaged neighborhoods are more likely to perpetrate violence against others because of the increased risk of victimization (and the resulting violent self-defense against that victimization), parental inability to counteract negative community influences, and lack of opportunities for success.

- Around 2 out of 10 high school girls were in a physical fight in the past year.
- Nine out of 100 high school girls missed at least one day of school in the past month because they didn't feel safe.

*Source: "Violence," Girlshealth.gov, Office on Women's Health (OWH), September 16, 2015.*

# Physical Fighting In Schools

Significant progress has been made in reducing physical fighting among adolescents. Since 1991, the percentage of high school students who had been in a physical fight at least once during the past 12 months decreased from 42 percent to 23 percent. However, nationwide, the percentage of students who had not gone to school because of safety concerns is still too high, with 6 percent of students missing at least 1 day of school because they felt they would be unsafe.

# Chapter 24
# Bullying

## What Is Bullying?

Bullying is when a person or a group shows unwanted aggression to another person who is not a sibling or a current dating partner. Cyberbullying (or "electronic aggression") is bullying that is done electronically, including through the Internet, e-mail, or mobile devices, among others.

Bullying can be:

- Physical: punching, beating, kicking, or pushing; stealing, hiding, or damaging another person's belongings; forcing someone to do things against his or her will

- Verbal: teasing, calling names, or insulting another person; threatening another person with physical harm; spreading rumors or untrue statements about another person

- Relational: refusing to talk to someone or making them feel left out; encouraging other individuals to bully someone

To be considered bullying, the behavior in question must be aggressive. The behavior must also involve an imbalance of power (e.g., physical strength, popularity, access to embarrassing details about a person) and be repetitive, meaning that it happens more than once or is highly likely to be repeated.

About This Chapter: Text beginning with the heading "What Is Bullying?" is excerpted from "Bullying," *Eunice Kennedy Shriver* National Institute of Child Health and Human Development (NICHD), January 28, 2014; Text beginning with the heading "What Is Cyberbullying?" is excerpted from "Cyberbullying," Girlshealth.gov, Office on Women's Health (OWH), April 15, 2014.

Bullying also includes cyberbullying and workplace bullying.

- Cyberbullying has increased with the increased use of the social media sites, the Internet, e-mail, and mobile devices. Unlike more traditional bullying, cyberbullying can be more anonymous and can occur nearly constantly. A person can be cyberbullied day or night, such as when they are checking their e-mail, using Facebook or another social network site, or even when they are using a mobile phone.

- Workplace bullying refers to adult behavior that is repeatedly aggressive and involves the use of power over another person at the workplace. Certain laws apply to adults in the workplace to help prevent such violence.

# Who Is Affected And How Many Are At Risk For Bullying?

- A survey from the National Center for Education Statistics (NCES) found that bullying continues to affect many school-aged children: nearly 1 out of 3 students in middle and high school reported that they were bullied at school. Among high school students, 1 out of 9 teens, or about 2.8 million, reported that they had been pushed, shoved, tripped, or spit on during the school year. In the same survey, another 1.5 million high school students reported that they had been threatened with physical harm, and 900,000 had been cyberbullied.

- Data from the 2011 Youth Risk Behavior Surveillance System from the Centers for Disease Control and Prevention (CDC) indicate that about 20 percent of U.S. students in grades 9 through 12 experienced bullying on school property.

- The National Center for Education Statistics (NCES) and Bureau of Justice Statistics (BJS) reported in their School Crime Supplement that about 28 percent of U.S. students in grades 6 through 12 experienced traditional bullying at school. Additionally, during the same school year, 6 percent of students reported being cyberbullied in other places besides at school.

# What Are Common Signs Of Being Bullied?

Signs of bullying include:

- Depression, loneliness, or anxiety
- Low self-esteem

- Headaches, stomachaches, tiredness, or poor eating habits

- Missing school, disliking school, or having poorer school performance than previously

- Self-destructive behaviors, such as running away from home or inflicting harm on oneself

- Thinking about suicide or attempting to commit suicide

- Unexplained injuries

- Lost or destroyed clothing, books, electronics, or jewelry

- Difficulty sleeping or frequent nightmares

- Sudden loss of friends or avoidance of social situations

# How Does Bullying Affect Health And Well-Being?

Bullying can lead to physical injury, social problems, emotional problems, and even death. Children and adolescents who are bullied are at increased risk for mental health problems, including depression, anxiety, headaches, and problems adjusting to school. Bullying also can cause long-term damage to self-esteem.

Children and adolescents who are bullies are at increased risk for substance use, academic problems, and violence to others later in life.

Children or adolescents who are both bullies and victims suffer the most serious effects of bullying and are at greater risk for mental and behavioral problems than those who are only bullied or who are only bullies.

*Eunice Kennedy Shriver* National Institute of Child Health and Human Development (NICHD) research studies show that anyone involved with bullying—those who bully others, those who are bullied, and those who bully and are bullied—are at increased risk for depression.

NICHD-funded research studies also found that unlike traditional forms of bullying, youth who are bullied electronically—such as by computer or cell phone—are at higher risk for depression than the youth who bully them. Even more surprising, the same studies found that cyber victims were at higher risk for depression than were cyberbullies or bully-victims (i.e., those who both bully others and are bullied themselves), which was not found in any other form of bullying.

# What Are Risk Factors For Being Bullied?

Children who are at risk of being bullied have one or more risk factors:

- Are seen as different from their peers (e.g., overweight, underweight, wear their hair differently, wear different clothing or wear glasses, or come from a different race/ethnicity)

- Are seen as weak or not able to defend themselves

- Are depressed, anxious, or have low self-esteem

- Have few friends or are less popular

- Do not socialize well with others

- Suffer from an intellectual or developmental disability

# What Can Be Done To Help Someone Who Is Being Bullied?

Support a child who is being bullied:

- You can listen to the child and let him or her know you are available to talk or even help. A child who is being bullied may struggle talking about it. Consider letting the child know there are other people who can talk with him or her about bullying. In addition, you might consider referring the child to a school counselor, psychologist, or other mental health specialist.

- Give the child advice about what he or she can do. You might want to include role-playing and acting out a bullying incident as you guide the child so that the child knows what to do in a real situation.

- Follow up with the child to show that you are committed to helping put a stop to the bullying.

Address the bullying behavior:

- Make sure a child whom you suspect or know is bullying knows what the problem behavior is and why it is not acceptable.

- Show kids that bullying is taken seriously. If you know someone is being a bully to someone else, tell the bully that bullying will not be tolerated. It is important, however, to demonstrate good behavior when speaking with a bully so that you serve as a role model of good interpersonal behavior.

If you feel that you have taken all possible steps to prevent bullying and nothing has worked, or someone is in immediate danger, there are other ways for you to help.

**Table 24.1.** Steps To Prevent Bullying

| The Problem | What You Can Do |
|---|---|
| A crime has occurred or someone is at immediate risk of harm. | Call 911. |
| Someone is feeling hopeless, helpless, or thinking of suicide. | Contact the National Suicide Prevention Lifeline External Web Site Policy online or at 1-800-273-TALK (1-800-273-8255). This toll-free call goes to the nearest crisis center in a national network. These centers provide crisis counseling and mental health referrals. |
| Someone is acting differently, such as sad or anxious, having trouble completing tasks, or not taking care of themselves. | Find a local counselor or other mental health services. |
| A child is being bullied in school. | Contact the:<br>• Teacher<br><br>• School counselor<br><br>• School coach<br><br>• School principal<br><br>• School superintendent<br><br>• Board of Education |
| Child is being bullied after school on the playground or in the neighborhood | • Neighborhood watch<br><br>• Playground security<br><br>• Team coach<br><br>• Local precinct/community police |
| The child's school is not addressing the bullying | Contact the:<br>• School superintendent<br><br>• Local Board of Education<br><br>• State Department of Education |

# What Is Cyberbullying?

Cyberbullying is hurting someone again and again using a computer, a cellphone, or another kind of electronic technology. Examples of cyberbullying include the following:

• Texting or emailing insults or nasty rumors about someone

- Posting mean comments about someone on Facebook, Twitter, and other social media sites

- Threatening someone through email or other technology

- Tricking someone into sharing embarrassing information

- Forwarding private text messages to hurt or embarrass someone

- Posting embarrassing photos or videos of someone

- Pretending to be someone else online to get that person in trouble or embarrass her

- Creating a website to make fun of someone

Teen girls say meanness lurks on social media. One out of 5 girls ages14 to 17 say people her age are mostly unkind to each other on social media. And one out of 3 girls ages 12 to 13 thought so.

Can you take a second to rewind and be kind before you post?

**Some teens think it's easier to get away with bullying online than in person.** Also, girls may be more likely to cyberbully than boys. Keep in mind that it's pretty easy to find out who has been cyberbullying. In fact, cyberbullies can get in a lot of trouble with their schools, and possibly even with the police.

**Cyberbullying hurts.** It can be easier to type something really mean than to say it to a person. But being cyberbullied can sometimes feel even worse than other kinds of bullying. That's because cyberbullying can come at you anytime, anywhere and can reach a lot of people.

Being cyberbullied can make you feel angry, afraid, helpless, and terribly sad. Also, teens who are cyberbullied are more likely than other teens to have problems such as using drugs, skipping school, and even getting sick.

**If you are being cyberbullied, talk to an adult you trust.** An adult can help you figure out how to handle the problem, and can offer you support.

**If you are cyberbullying, it's time to stop.** You are not only hurting someone else, you could hurt yourself. You can lose friends and get in trouble with your school or even with the police. If you can't seem to stop yourself from cyberbullying, get help from an adult you trust.

**You may hurt someone online without really meaning to do it.** It may seem funny to vote for the ugliest kid in school, for example, but try to think about how that person feels. And if you get a message that makes you mad, go away and come back before writing something you may regret. Nearly half of teenage cellphone users say they regretted a text message they sent. Remember, nothing is really secret or private on the Internet, and things you post online can stay there forever.

# How To Prevent Cyberbullying?

Here are some tips that may help protect you from being cyberbullied:

- Don't give out your passwords or personal information. Even your friends could wind up giving your passwords to someone who shouldn't have them.

- Use the privacy options on social networking sites like Facebook, Instagram, and Tumblr that let you choose who can see what you post.

- Don't friend people online if you don't know them, even if you have friends in common.

- Be careful about what you write or what images you send or post because nothing is really private on the Internet.

- If you are using a site like Facebook on a computer in the library, log out before you walk away. If you don't log out, the next person who uses the computer could get into your account.

# If You Are Cyberbullied

If you are cyberbullied, you can get help. Here are some important tips:

- If someone bullies you, don't respond. Bullies are looking for a reaction, and you may be able to stop the bullying if you ignore or block the person.

- Save any evidence of cyberbullying, print it out, and show it to a trusted adult.

- Use options that let you block email, cellphone, and text messages from a cyberbully. You can also stop a person from seeing your Facebook information. If you need help, ask an adult, your cellphone company, or the website where you want to block someone.

- If you are being cyberbullied, ask if your school can get involved.

- Report bullying to your Internet service provider, phone company, email provider, or the website where it happened. Sites like Twitter, YouTube, and Instagram have online forms for reporting.

- Report cyberbullying to police if it involves threats of violence or pornography.

Sometimes, teens don't want to tell their parents that they are being cyberbullied because they are afraid their parents will take away their phone or computer. If you have this concern, tell your parents, and work with them to figure out a solution. The most important thing is for you to be safe.

# Sexting And Cyberbullying

Sexting is sending naked or partly naked photos to someone online or by cellphone. Sometimes, a guy may pressure you to send these kinds of photos. Sometimes, friends may dare you to do it.

It's a very bad idea to send nude photos or forward someone else's. Messages can be traced back to you, and photos can quickly get forwarded to a lot of people. You can really hurt someone's feelings or your own reputation. You can even get in legal trouble for forwarding something that could be considered child pornography.

# Examples Of Cyberbullying

Unfortunately, there are lots of ways to hurt someone through technology. Below are some examples.

- **Love, who?**

  Laurie watched as Emma logged on to her account so she could get Emma's password. Later, Laurie logged on as Emma and sent a mean message to Emma's best friend.

- **Picture this!**

  Sue, an overweight high schooler, was changing in the locker room after gym class. Annabelle snapped a pic of Sue with her phone and sent it all around school.

- **Privacy, please!**

  Karen pretended to be Mara's friend and sent her a message asking lots of questions. Mara replied with some really personal info. Karen shared what she said and added her own comment, "Mara is a loser!"

- **Breakup breakdown.**

  After Sarah broke up with Dave, he started texting her constantly at all times of the day and night.

# Chapter 25
# Hazing

## Overview[1]

We all want to belong. Whether it's to the chess club or the football team or a sorority or fraternity, belonging to a group of people who are bonded together gives us the feeling that we aren't alone. In high school, and especially in college when people leave their hometowns and are trying to fit in to a new environment, these clubs can feel like a lifeline. And for many people, these groups become like family—you can be a "Sorority Sister" and "Fraternity Brother."

But what's the cost of joining? All too often, it's going through an embarrassing and potentially dangerous initiation ritual—known as hazing.

## Suspect Hazing?[1]

Hazing can often be confidentially reported to school officials. There is also a national, toll-free, anti-hazing hotline at 1-888-NOT-HAZE (1-888-668-4293). Not sure if it's hazing? Call anyway. Ask yourself whether you would tell a potential member about the activity before they joined.

## What Is Hazing?[1]

Basically, hazing is when an organized group participates in activities that involves harassment, humiliation, and/or physical and emotional abuse as a way of letting someone join their

About This Chapter: This chapter contains text excerpted from documents published by two public domain sources. Text under headings marked 1 are excerpted from "Hazing And Alcohol: Time To Break With Tradition," NIDA for Teens, National Institute on Drug Abuse (NIDA), April 10, 2015; Text under headings marked 2 are excerpted from "Hazing Versus Bullying," Office on Women's Health (OWH), U.S. Department of Health and Human Services (HHS), April 15, 2014.

club, team, organization, etc. Hazing can be violent and it can cause serious physical harm, including death in extreme cases. Some common forms of hazing include:

- Drinking games (which often involve having people drink a lot of alcohol very quickly)

- Sleep deprivation, kidnapping, beating a person up, or sexual abuse

- Enduring harsh weather without proper clothing

- Branding, tattooing, or piercing

- Walking a "gauntlet" of people who have battering sticks and weapons

More than 50 percent of college students and 47 percent of high school students involved in clubs, teams, and organizations experience hazing. It's passed down from class to class. The hazed become the hazers and the cycle of bad behavior continues.

Since 1970, at least one college student dies in the United States each year because of an initiation gone wrong. Studies have found that, in college, making people drink too much alcohol is the most common form of hazing. Alcohol also makes it easier to haze. Being drunk helps current members feel less bad about abusing the new pledges.

## What Are Warning Signs Of Hazing?[2]

Here are some possible signs of hazing:

- You have heard from friends about a group using hazing.
- You feel a knot in your stomach—trust your instincts!
- You have been warned by teachers or other adults that the group is dangerous.
- You have seen the group push others to do things that you believe are wrong or dangerous.
- You feel afraid to break away from the group.
- The group leaders are very mean.
- The group leaders do things that don't seem right and then make you promise not to tell anyone.

## What Can I Do To Stay Safe From Hazing?[2]

If you are concerned about hazing, try to find out if a group is known for having mean rituals. If you think you are going a place where you might be hazed, have a plan to stay safe. Stick together with friends you trust, and make sure you have a way to get home safely.

If you are being hazed, tell an adult. Some states have laws against hazing. Remember, no one has a right to hurt you or pressure you to do something that feels wrong!

# Immediate Care Of Someone Who Has Passed Out[1]

Check four "PUBS" signs to determine if the situation is an emergency:

- Puking (while passed out)

- Unresponsive to stimulation (pinch or shake)

- Breathing (slow, shallow, or no breathing)

- Skin (blue, cold, or clammy)

If even one of these signs is present, call 911. Do not wait—call 911.

And never leave someone alone to "sleep it off." If someone has passed out, they have had a dangerous amount of alcohol and they should be monitored to make sure none of the symptoms mentioned occur.

Alcohol is also one of the ways people die from hazing. It's what killed 18-year-old college freshman Lynn Gordon Bailey ("Gordie"). He participated in a hazing ritual that involved drinking too much alcohol, and 3 weeks into his first year at college, he died from that ritual. Gordie wasn't a small guy—he was an athlete. Probably no one would have thought when they looked at him that he would die from drinking too much. But no matter how fit you are, if you drink too much alcohol too quickly for your body to process, your vital organs can shut down, and you can die. Hearing Gordie's story may help people to think about what could have been done differently.

# So What's A Person To Do?[1]

There's no shame in saying no or standing up for yourself—but it's usually easier to do before the hazing begins. Learn as much as you can about the pledging process for the group you want to join. Know that not every club, group, or house is going to ask you to do the same things. While it's true that most people survive the pledging or initiation process, it's equally true that for some people, the beatings or binge drinking have led to deaths.

Ideally, you'll find a group whose initiation isn't about humiliation. After all, do you really want to be part of a group that purposely hurts new members? Or tries to make them physically sick? Or that has racist chants? Or sexist websites?

Team building and other bonding exercises don't have to be negative. Lots of groups organize other activities that people have to do to join the group—but it doesn't cost them their dignity or risk their health or wellbeing. These include:

- Doing community service

- Going out for group events

- Playing recreational games/sports

- Organizing a fundraising event

- Completing a ropes course, leadership courses, or other similar activities

- Tutoring or mentoring

This list goes on and on—because there are always better alternatives to bullying, or hazing, or any form of abuse. And maybe it's been a "tradition" to be hurtful and hateful—but we are not alone in thinking that it is time to break these traditions.

# Chapter 26
# Youth Gangs

## What Is A Gang?

There is no universally agreed-upon definition of "gang" in the United States. Gang, youth gang, and street gang are terms widely and often interchangeably used in mainstream coverage. Reference to gangs often implies youth gangs. In some cases, youth gangs are distinguished from other types of gangs; how youth is defined may vary as well.

Motorcycle gangs, prison gangs, hate groups, adult organized crime groups, terrorist organizations, and other types of security threat groups are frequently but not always treated separately from gangs in both practice and research.

> The prevalence of youth under 18 in gangs is higher in smaller cities and rural communities where gang problems are less established, compared to larger cities.
>
> *Source: "Federal Data," Youth.gov, March 6, 2013.*

## Defining "Youth Gangs"

The National Gang Center (which is cosponsored by the Bureau of Justice Assistance and the Office of Juvenile Justice and Delinquency Prevention) conducts the National Youth Gang

About This Chapter: Text under the heading "What Is Gang?" is excerpted from "Gangs And Gang Crime," National Institute of Justice (NIJ), U.S. Department of Justice (DOJ), October 28, 2011. Reviewed November 2016; Text under the heading "Risk And Protective Factors" is excerpted from "Risk And Protective Factors," Youth.gov, March 6, 2013. Reviewed November 2016; Text beginning with the heading "Effects Of Youth Involved In Gangs" is excerpted from "Adverse Effects," Youth.gov, March 6, 2013. Reviewed November 2016.

Survey. The survey reports solely on youth gangs, which the National Gang Center describes as "a group of youths or young adults [the responding agency is] willing to identify as a 'gang.'"

When they report to the National Youth Gang Survey, law enforcement agencies indicate that group criminality is of greatest importance in how they define a gang. The presence of leadership is of least importance.

Much of the research literature about gangs focuses primarily on youth gangs, as opposed to adult gangs. Researchers accept the following criteria for classifying groups as gangs:

- The group has three or more members, generally aged 12–24.

- Members share an identity, typically linked to a name, and often other symbols.

- Members view themselves as a gang, and they are recognized by others as a gang.

- The group has some permanence and a degree of organization.

- The group is involved in an elevated level of criminal activity.

## Defining "Types" Of Gangs

The National Gang Intelligence Center and the National Drug Intelligence Center collaborated to produce the *National Gang Threat Assessment* in 2009. The book discusses street gangs, prison gangs and outlaw motorcycle gangs. Each gang type merits its own definition and discussion of the characteristics that differ at national, regional and local levels.

## Defining "Gang Member" And "Gang Crime"

Localities interested in pursuing anti-gang policies, strategies and programs face the challenge of developing operational definitions for the terms "gang," "gang member" and "gang crime" (or "gang-related offense"). Many criminal justice policymakers and practitioners operate under practical definitions unique to their locality and its explicit gang-related challenges.

Some localities fail to address the need for definition or to consider elements of definitions already in use. Failing to define the terms "gang" and "gang crime" as the terms are commonly used in a community undermines the community's ability to reliably measure progress and outcomes related to gangs and gang activity.

California and other states and localities have instituted various criteria and threshold levels an offender must meet to be classified as a gang member. Multiple criteria may need to be documented.

For example,

1. a reliable source must identify the offender as a gang member, and

2. the offender must display gang symbols or use hand signs and display gang tattoos.

# Risk And Protective Factors

The risk and protective factors of youth gang involvement can span multiple domains from the individual level (aggressiveness) to the peer (delinquent siblings), school (academic failure), and community levels (poverty). Risk factors encourage or increase the likelihood of youth participating in gangs; whereas a protective factor acts as a buffer in the presence of risk factors. Proper assessment of risk and protective factors for youth and gang involvement helps to inform the development and implementation of prevention and intervention strategies.

Most youth who become affiliated with gangs lack positive supports from parents, schools, peers, and community. Research also indicates a close link between gang involvement and delinquent activity such as substance use. Findings indicate that youth who engage in delinquent activities, specifically illicit alcohol and drug use, are more likely to join gangs and that, as a result of gang involvement, youth are more likely to use illicit drugs and alcohol.

Risk factors that significantly affect a youth's chance for gang-involvement include the following:

- Aggressiveness
- Early initiation of violent behavior
- Parental criminality
- Child maltreatment
- Low levels of parental involvement
- Parent-child separation
- Academic failure
- Lack of school connectedness
- Truancy and school dropout
- Frequent school transitions
- Delinquent siblings and peers
- Peer gang membership

- Poverty

- Substance use (e.g., illicit drugs and alcohol)

- Community disorganization

- Availability of drugs and firearms

- Exposure to violence and racial prejudice

Research suggests that the greater the number of risk factors that a youth experiences, the more likely he or she is to join a gang. It also shows that a youth's risk for gang involvement significantly increases as he or she accrues more than two risk factors. Therefore, prevention programs that target risk factors can help mitigate youth gang involvement. Additionally, efforts to minimize youth gang involvement can be addressed through promoting protective factors. Research suggests that as youth accumulate more protective factors it lowers the risk of gang involvement.

Protective factors that have been identified as influential to youth gang involvement include:

- Parental involvement and monitoring

- Family support

- Coping skills (interpersonal skills)

- Positive social connections

- Peer support

- Academic achievement

- Reducing delinquency, alcohol, and drug use

# Effects Of Youth Involved In Gangs

The numerous consequences stemming from gang involvement can have varying degrees of short and long-term negative outcomes. Youth who become involved in gangs face the increased risk of

- dropping out of school

- teen parenthood

- unemployment

- victimization

- drug and alcohol abuse

- committing petty and violent crimes and

- juvenile conviction and incarceration

Further, a youth's involvement with a gang (or gangs) also leads to an increased likelihood of economic hardship and family problems in adulthood, which in turn, contribute to involvement in street crime and/or arrest in adulthood. Research has suggested that the longer an adolescent stays in a gang the more disruption he or she will experience while transitioning into adulthood and in adulthood itself.

# Impact On Communities

Large communities, those with a population over 50,000, are at the greatest risk of significant gang activity, and community members face heightened fear that they, their families, schools, or businesses, will become victims of theft and/or violence. Further, communities with gang activity are disproportionately affected by theft, negative economic impact, vandalism, assault, gun violence, illegal drug trade, and homicide.

# Impact On Society

On the societal level, youth gang involvement costs local, state, and federal governments a substantial amount of money in prevention, response, incarceration, and rehabilitation efforts. It has been estimated that overall crime in the United States costs taxpayers $655 billion annually with a substantial amount of this crime attributed to gang activity.

# Chapter 27

# Hate Crimes

## What Are Hate Crimes?

Hate crimes are the highest priority of the Federal Bureau of Investigation's (FBI) Civil Rights program, not only because of the devastating impact they have on families and communities, but also because groups that preach hatred and intolerance can plant the seed of terrorism here in our country. The Bureau investigates hundreds of these cases every year and works to detect and deter further incidents through law enforcement training, public outreach, and partnerships with a myriad of community groups.

Traditionally, FBI investigations of hate crimes were limited to crimes in which the perpetrators acted based on a bias against the victim's race, color, religion, or national origin. In addition, investigations were restricted to those wherein the victim was engaged in a federally protected activity. With the passage of the Matthew Shepard and James Byrd, Jr., Hate Crimes Prevention Act of 2009, the Bureau became authorized to investigate these crimes without this prohibition. This landmark legislation also expanded the role of the FBI to allow for the investigation of hate crimes committed against those based on biases of actual or perceived sexual orientation, gender identity, disability, or gender.

About This Chapter: Text beginning with the heading "What Are Hate Crimes" is excerpted from "What Are Hate Crimes," Federal Bureau of Investigation (FBI), U.S. Department of Justice (DOJ), June 18, 2006. Reviewed November 2016; Text beginning with the heading "What Motivates Hate Offenders" is excerpted from "Hate Crime," National Institute of Justice (NIJ), December 22, 2010, Reviewed November 2016; Text beginning with the heading "Victims" is excerpted from "2014 Hate Crime Statistics," Federal Bureau of Investigation (FBI), U.S. Department of Justice (DOJ), 2014.

## Defining A Hate Crime

A hate crime is a traditional offense like murder, arson, or vandalism with an added element of bias. For the purposes of collecting statistics, the FBI has defined a hate crime as a "criminal offense against a person or property motivated in whole or in part by an offender's bias against a race, religion, disability, sexual orientation, ethnicity, gender, or gender identity." Hate itself is not a crime—and the FBI is mindful of protecting freedom of speech and other civil liberties.

These efforts serve as a backstop for investigations by state and local authorities, which handle the vast majority of hate crime cases throughout the country.

## What Motivates Hate Offenders?

According to the Bureau of Justice Statistics, race is the most common motivating factor in hate crime offending reported to the police (61%), followed by religion (14%), sexual orientation (13%), ethnicity (11%), and victim disability (1%). In racially motivated offenses, 60 percent targeted blacks and 30 percent targeted whites.

One study classified hate crime offenders into four categories that differ with respect to the psychological and situational factors that lead to hate crime offending. This typology is widely used by law enforcement for training officers in the investigation and identification of hate crime.

## Response To Hate Crimes

Responses to hate crime range from changes in legislation to law enforcement training aimed at improving responses to these crimes; to investigation, prosecution, and prevention of hate crimes; to victim support programs; to diversity and tolerance education programs. Most States and metropolitan areas have some form of government-sponsored hate crime initiative involving criminal justice agencies. Municipal police departments in many large urban areas have hate crime units within their department, and police departments are often involved as members of State or regional hate crime task forces.

The Federal Government has also supported several initiatives to address hate crime. The Bureau of Justice Assistance (BJA), for example, has provided funding for the Center for the Prevention of Hate Violence at the University of Southern Maine to produce a series of reports on BJA-supported initiatives and State and local demonstration projects. Many recommendations and "best practice" suggestions for how to effectively address, prevent, and respond to hate crime have emerged over the past 15 years. Although these recommendations are derived from practical experience and expert opinion and appear well-conceived, none of the myriad criminal justice responses has been subjected to rigorous empirical evaluation.

# Victims

In the Uniform Crime Reporting (UCR) Program, the victim of a hate crime may be an individual, a business, an institution, or society as a whole. In 2014, the nation's law enforcement agencies reported that there were 6,727 victims of hate crimes. Of these victims, 46 were victimized in 17 separate multiple-bias incidents.

In 2013, the national UCR Program began collecting revised race and ethnicity data in accordance with a directive from the U.S. Government's Office of Management and Budget. The race categories were expanded from four (White, Black, American Indian or Alaska Native, and Asian or Other Pacific Islander) to five (White, Black or African American, American Indian or Alaska Native, Asian, and Native Hawaiian or Other Pacific Islander). The ethnicity categories changed from "Hispanic" and "Non-Hispanic" to "Hispanic or Latino" and "Not Hispanic or Latino."

## By Bias Motivation

An analysis of data for victims of single-bias hate crime incidents showed that:

- 48.3 percent of the victims were targeted because of the offenders' bias against race.

- 18.7 percent were targeted because of bias against sexual orientation.

- 17.1 percent were victimized because of bias against religion.

- 12.3 percent were victimized because of bias against ethnicity.

- 1.6 percent were victims of gender-identity bias.

- 1.4 percent were targeted because of bias against disability.

- 0.6 percent (40 individuals) were victims of gender bias.

Further examination of these bias categories showed the following details:

### Racial Bias

Among single-bias hate crime incidents in 2014, there were 3,227 victims of racially motivated hate crime.

- 62.7 percent were victims of crimes motivated by their offenders' anti-Black or African American bias.

- 22.7 percent were victims of anti-White bias.

- 6.2 percent were victims of anti-Asian bias.

- 4.6 percent were victims of anti-American Indian or Alaska Native bias.

- 3.7 percent were victims of bias against a group of individuals in which more than one race was represented (anti-multiple races, group).

- 0.1 percent (4 individuals) were victims of anti-Native Hawaiian or Other Pacific Islander bias.

## Sexual-Orientation Bias

Of the 1,248 victims targeted due to sexual-orientation bias:

- 56.3 percent were victims of crimes motivated by their offenders' anti-gay (male) bias.

- 24.4 percent were victims of anti-lesbian, gay, bisexual, or transgender (mixed group) bias.

- 13.9 percent were victims of anti-lesbian bias.

- 3.8 percent were victims of anti-bisexual bias.

- 1.5 percent were victims of anti-heterosexual bias.

## Religious Bias

Of the 1,140 victims of anti-religious hate crimes:

- 56.8 percent were victims of crimes motivated by their offenders' anti-Jewish bias.

- 16.1 percent were victims of anti-Islamic (Muslim) bias.

- 6.2 percent were victims of bias against groups of individuals of varying religions (anti-multiple religions, group).

- 6.1 percent were victims of anti-Catholic bias.

- 2.5 percent were victims of anti-Protestant bias.

- 1.2 percent were victims of anti-Atheist/Agnostic bias.

- 11.0 percent were victims of bias against other religions (anti-other religion).

## Ethnicity

Hate crimes motivated by the offenders' biases toward particular ethnicities were directed at 821 victims. Of these victims:

- 52.6 percent were victimized because of anti-not Hispanic or Latino bias.

- 47.4 percent were targeted because of anti-Hispanic or Latino bias.

## Disability Bias

Of the 96 victims of hate crimes due to the offenders' biases against disabilities:

- 70 were targets of anti-mental disability bias.

- 26 were victims of anti-physical disability bias.

## Gender Bias

Of the 40 victims of hate crime motivated by offenders' biases toward gender:

- 28 were categorized as anti-female.

- 12 were anti-male.

## Gender-Identity Bias

Of the 109 victims of gender-identity bias:

- 69 were victims of anti-transgender bias.

- 40 were victims of anti-gender non-conforming bias.

## By Crime Category

Of the 6,727 victims of hate crime, 60.2 percent were victims of crimes against persons, and 39.0 percent were victims of crimes against property. The remaining 0.8 percent were victims of crimes against society.

## By Offense Type

### Crimes Against Persons

In 2014, 4,048 victims of hate crimes were victims of crimes against persons. Regarding these victims and the crimes committed against them:

- 4 persons were murdered, and 9 were raped. (Concerning rape, data for all 9 rapes were submitted under the UCR Program's revised definition.)

- 43.1 percent of the victims were intimidated.

- 37.4 percent were victims of simple assault.

- 19.0 percent were victims of aggravated assault.

- 0.1 percent (6) were victims of other types of offenses, which are collected only in the National Incident-Based Reporting System (NIBRS).

## Crimes Against Property

In 2014, 2,624 victims of hate crimes were victims of crimes against property. Of these:

- 72.7 percent were victims of destruction/damage/vandalism.

- 9.8 percent were victims of larceny-theft.

- 7.9 percent were victims of burglary.

- 5.3 percent were victims of robbery.

- 1.5 percent were victims of arson.

- 0.8 percent (22) were victims of motor vehicle theft.

- 2.1 percent were victims of other types of hate crime offenses, which are collected only in the NIBRS.

## Crimes Against Society

There were 55 victims of hate crimes categorized as crimes against society. Crimes against society (e.g., weapon law violations, drug/narcotic offenses, gambling offenses) represent society's prohibition against engaging in certain types of activity; they are typically victimless crimes in which property is not the object.

# Offenders

Law enforcement agencies that reported hate crime data to the Uniform Crime Reporting (UCR) Program identified 5,192 known offenders in 5,479 bias-motivated incidents in 2014. In the UCR Program, the term known offender does not imply that the suspect's identity is known; rather, the term indicates that some aspect of the suspect was identified, thus distinguishing the suspect from an unknown offender. Law enforcement agencies specify the number of offenders and, when possible, the race, ethnicity, and age of the offender or offenders as a group.

## By Race, Ethnicity, And Age

### Race

In 2014, race was reported for 5,192 known hate crime offenders. Of these offenders:

- 52.0 percent were White.

- 23.2 percent were Black or African American.

- 6.9 percent were groups made up of individuals of various races (group of multiple races).

- 1.1 percent (58 offenders) were American Indian or Alaska Native.

- 0.8 percent (39 offenders) were Asian.

- Less than 0.1 percent (2 offenders) were Native Hawaiian or Other Pacific Islander.

- 16.0 percent were unknown.

## Ethnicity

The ethnicity was reported for 975 known hate crime offenders. Of these:

- 47.6 percent were in the ethnic category Not Hispanic or Latino.

- 6.5 percent were Hispanic or Latino.

- 1.7 percent were groups made up of individuals of various ethnicities (group of multiple ethnicities).

- 44.2 percent were of unknown ethnicity.

## Age

Age was reported for 1,875 known hate crime offenders. Of these:

- 81.0 percent were 18 and over.

- 19.0 percent were under 18.

## By Crime Category

### Crimes Against Persons

A total of 3,925 known hate crime offenders committed crimes against persons in 2014. Of these offenders:

- 42.4 percent committed simple assault.

- 34.0 percent intimidated their victims.

- 22.9 percent committed aggravated assault.

- 0.3 percent (10 offenders) raped their victims.

- 0.1 percent (5 offenders) murdered their victims.

- 0.3 percent (11 offenders) committed other types of offenses, which are collected only in the UCR Program's National Incident-Based Reporting System (NIBRS).

## Crimes Against Property

A total of 1,455 known hate crime offenders committed crimes against property in 2014. Of these offenders:

- 54.4 percent committed destruction/damage/vandalism.

- 17.5 percent committed robbery.

- 12.7 percent committed burglary.

- 10.4 percent committed larceny-theft.

- 1.4 percent committed arson.

- 1.0 percent (15 offenders) committed motor vehicle theft.

- 2.5 percent committed other types of offenses, which are collected only in the NIBRS.

## Crimes Against Society

In 2014, 61 known offenders committed 53 crimes against society involving 55 victims. Crimes against society are collected only via the NIBRS. Crimes against society (e.g., weapon law violations, drug/narcotic offenses, gambling offenses) represent society's prohibition against engaging in certain types of activity; they are typically victimless crimes in which property is not the object.

# Chapter 28

# School Violence And Effects Of School Violence Exposure

In the United States, an estimated 50 million students are enrolled in pre-kindergarten through 12th grade. Another 15 million students attend colleges and universities across the country. While U.S. schools remain relatively safe, any amount of violence is unacceptable. Parents, teachers, and administrators expect schools to be safe havens of learning. Acts of violence can disrupt the learning process and have a negative effect on students, the school itself, and the broader community.

## What Is School Violence?

School violence is a subset of youth violence, a broader public health problem. Violence is the intentional use of physical force or power, against another person, group, or community, with the behavior likely to cause physical or psychological harm. Youth violence typically includes persons between the ages of 10 and 24, although pathways to youth violence can begin in early childhood.

**Examples of violent behavior include:**

- Bullying

- Fighting (e.g., punching, slapping, kicking)

- Weapon use

- Electronic aggression

- Gang violence

About This Chapter: Text in this chapter begins with excerpts from "About School Violence," Centers for Disease Control and Prevention (CDC), September 22, 2016; Text beginning with the heading "Why Is School Violence A Public Health Problem" is excerpted from "Understanding School Violence," Centers for Disease Control and Prevention (CDC), 2016.

**School violence occurs:**

- On school property

- On the way to or from school

- During a school-sponsored event

- On the way to or from a school-sponsored event

# Why Is School Violence A Public Health Problem?

School associated violent deaths are rare.

- 31 homicides of school-age youth, ages 5 to 18 years, occurred at school during the 2012–2013 school year.

- Of all youth homicides, less than 2.6 percent occur at school, and this percentage has been relatively stable for the past decade.

In 2014, there were about 486,400 nonfatal violent victimizations at school among students 12 to 18 years of age.

Approximately 9 percent of teachers report that they have been threatened with injury by a student from their school; 5 percent of school teachers reported that they had been physically attacked by a student from their school.

In 2013, 12 percent of students ages 12–18 reported that gangs were present at their school during the school year.

In a 2015 nationally representative sample of youth in grades 9–12:

- 7.8 percent reported being in a physical fight on school property in the 12 months before the survey.

- 5.6 percent reported that they did not go to school on one or more days in the 30 days before the survey because they felt unsafe at school or on their way to or from school.

- 4.1 percent reported carrying a weapon (gun, knife or club) on school property on one or more days in the 30 days before the survey.

- 6 percent reported being threatened or injured with a weapon on school property one or more times in the 12 months before the survey.

- 20.2 percent reported being bullied on school property and 15.5 percent reported being bullied electronically during the 12 months before the survey.

# How Does School Violence Affect Health?

Deaths resulting from school violence are only part of the problem. Many young people experience nonfatal injuries. Some of these injuries are relatively minor and include cuts, bruises, and broken bones. Other injuries, like gunshot wounds and head trauma, are more serious and can lead to permanent disability.

Not all injuries are visible. Exposure to youth violence and school violence can lead to a wide array of negative health behaviors and outcomes, including alcohol and drug use and suicide. Depression, anxiety, and many other psychological problems, including fear, can result from school violence.

# Who Is At Risk For School Violence?

A number of factors can increase the risk of a youth engaging in violence at school. However, the presence of these factors does not always mean that a young person will become an offender.

Risk factors for school and youth violence include:

- prior history of violence
- drug, alcohol, or tobacco use
- association with delinquent peers
- poor family functioning
- poor grades in school
- poverty in the community

# How Can We Prevent School Violence?

The goal is to stop school violence from happening in the first place. Several prevention strategies have been identified.

- Universal, school-based prevention programs can significantly lower rates of aggression and violent behavior. These programs are delivered to all students in a school or grade level. They teach about various topics and develop skills, such as emotional self-awareness and control, positive social skills, problem solving, conflict resolution, and teamwork.

- Parent- and family-based programs can improve family relations and lower the risk for violence by children especially when the programs are started early. These programs provide parents with education about child development and teach skills to communicate and solve problems in nonviolent ways.

- Street outreach programs can significantly reduce youth violence. These programs connect trained staff with at-risk youth to conduct conflict mediation, make service referrals, and change beliefs about the acceptability of violence.

# Chapter 29

# Teen Firearm Violence

## How Prevalent Is Gun Violence In America?

According to the National Crime Victimization Survey (NCVS), 467,321 persons were victims of a crime committed with a firearm in 2011. In the same year, data collected by the Federal Bureau of Investigation (FBI) show that firearms were used in 68 percent of murders, 41 percent of robbery offenses and 21 percent of aggravated assaults nationwide.

Most homicides in the United States are committed with firearms, especially handguns.

Community Violence Prevention Strategies such as Baltimore's Safe Streets program, a street-level outreach and conflict mediation strategy, resulted in fewer homicides and non-fatal shootings in most implementation communities and less acceptance to use violence to solve conflicts.

*Source: "Understanding And Preventing Violence," Centers for Disease Control and Prevention (CDC), 2013.*

## Gangs And Gun-Related Homicide

Gun-related homicide is most prevalent among gangs and during the commission of felony crimes. In 1980, the percentage of homicides caused by firearms during arguments was about the same as from gang involvement (about 70 percent), but by 1993, nearly all gang-related homicides involved guns (95 percent), whereas the percentage of gun homicides related to arguments remained relatively constant. The percentage of gang-related homicides caused by

About This Chapter: This chapter includes text excerpted from "Gun Violence," National Institute of Justice (NIJ), U.S. Department of Justice (DOJ), April 4, 2013. Reviewed November 2016.

guns fell slightly to 92 percent in 2008, but the percentage of homicides caused by firearms during the commission of a felony rose from about 60 percent to about 74 percent from 1980 to 2005.

## Nonfatal Firearm-Related Crime

Nonfatal firearm-related crime has fallen significantly in recent years, from almost 1.3 million incidents in 1994 to a low of 331,618 incidents in 2008. Since then it has risen; in 2011 there were 414,562 incidents.

As a percentage of all violent incidents (i.e., rape, sexual assault, robbery and aggravated assault), between 1993 and 2011, nonfatal gun crime has ranged from a high of 8 percent to a low of 5 percent. In 2011, firearm crimes comprised 8 percent of all violent crimes.

## Who Has Guns And How Are They Acquired?

National Institute of Justice's (NIJ) earliest firearms studies uncovered who owns guns, legally and illegally, and how illegal gun trafficking is tied to juvenile gun violence and other crimes such as drug dealing and gang crime. Highlights of these studies:

- Many juveniles and young adults can easily obtain guns illegally; most claim to carry them for self-defense.

- A study of persons arrested for a wide range of crimes showed that a higher percentage of arrestees than regular citizens own firearms. Arrestees are also more likely to be injured or killed by gun violence. Within a community, this amounts to an identifiable group of "career" offenders.

- Surveys of offenders have found that they prefer newer, high-quality guns and may steal or borrow them; most, however, acquire guns "off the street" through the illicit gun market.

## Who Is Most Affected By Gun Violence?

People between the ages of 15 and 24 are most likely to be targeted by gun violence as opposed to other forms of violence. From 1976 to 2005, 77 percent of homicide victims ages 15–17 died from gun-related injuries. This age group was most at risk for gun violence during this time period.

Teens and young adults are more likely than persons of other ages to be murdered with a gun. Most violent gun crime, especially homicide, occurs in cities and urban communities.

Intimate partner violence can be fatal when a gun is involved—**from 1990 to 2005, two-thirds of spouse and ex-spouse homicide victims were killed by guns.** The overall number of firearm homicides among intimates has fallen considerably during the past 30 years, however.

# Gun Violence Prevention

Faced with a national epidemic of gun violence that began in the 1980s and continued throughout most of the 1990s, the federal government launched a new effort to help local authorities address gun crime. Many cities worked with (NIJ) researchers and other federal, state and local partners to design and test interventions to get illegally obtained guns off the streets and out of the hands of urban youth.

Initially, firearms violence intervention and research focused on either reducing the **demand** for illegally obtained guns or reducing the **supply**. More than 20 years of intervention programs, however, have shown that a single approach is not likely to work. To reduce gun violence, a sustained program that addresses both demand and supply is needed. A successful intervention will have elements of federal-local law enforcement collaboration, community involvement, targeted intervention tactics and continuous program evaluation.

A key lesson learned from several decades of gun violence intervention programs is that sustained federal-local partnerships improve efforts to reduce gun violence within a city or community. The U.S. Department of Justice's (DOJ) national gun violence reduction program, **Project Safe Neighborhoods**, helps localities develop and implement partnerships and strategies that are likely to work.

# Chapter 30
# Terrorism

Terrorism is a violent act committed by people who want to get attention for their cause. When a terrorist strikes, it seems like the entire world is upside down and confusing. It's hard to believe what's happened or that someone would do something like that.

Acts of terrorism have been a reality in many places for years. In the United States, the worst attacks happened on September 11, 2001. In the years that followed, other attacks also happened in Spain, London, and elsewhere.

Terrorism scares everyone because no one knows when or where it will take place. So how do you cope with it all? Here are some things you can do:

- **Give yourself a fear reality check.** It's normal to be worried about your safety and your family's safety. Even though your chances of being in an attack are very, very small, the images you see on TV or online make terrorist attacks seem close by.

- **Share your feelings.** Anger, sadness, fear, and numbness are some of the reactions you might have. Don't be embarrassed or afraid to express how you feel. Just talking and sharing your feelings with your parents, friends, teachers, and others can help them and help you.

- **Take care of yourself.** Losing sleep, not eating, and worrying too much can make you sick. As much as possible, try to get enough sleep, eat right, exercise, and keep a normal routine. It may be hard to do, but it can keep you healthy and better able to handle a tough time.

About This Chapter: Text in this chapter begins with excerpts from "Terrorism," © 1995–2016. The Nemours Foundation/KidsHealth®. Reprinted with permission; Text under the heading "Definitions Of Terrorism" is excerpted from "Terrorism," National Institute of Justice (NIJ), September 13, 2011. Reviewed November 2016. Text under the heading "How To Help Prevent Terrorist Attacks" is excerpted from "Terrorism," Federal Bureau of Investigation (FBI), 2006. Reviewed November 2016.

- **Limit the time you spend watching the news.** It's good to be informed about what's happening, but spending hours watching the news reports can make you feel more anxious and sad.

- **Be respectful of others.** You may have heard certain countries, religions, or political causes blamed for terrorism. But very few people believe in killing and hurting innocent people to make their point. Don't give into prejudice by blaming a whole group, or disliking people just because of the country where they were born, the faith they practice, the way they dress, or the color of their skin.

- **Join with others.** Participating in candlelight vigils, religious ceremonies, memorial services, or other events can be helpful. It's a way to show you care and that the community is sticking together during a sad time.

- **Get additional support.** A traumatic event can cause strong reactions, but if your feelings make it impossible for you to function and do normal stuff, like go to school, it's time to seek additional help. Turn to a parent, teacher, religious leader, or guidance counselor, so you can get the help you need.

# Definitions Of Terrorism

The search for a universal, precise definition of terrorism has been challenging for researchers and practitioners alike. Different definitions exist across the federal, international and research communities.

Title 22 of the U.S. Code, Section 2656f(d) defines terrorism as "premeditated, politically motivated violence perpetrated against noncombatant targets by subnational groups or clandestine agents, usually intended to influence an audience."

The Federal Bureau of Investigation (FBI) defines terrorism as "the unlawful use of force or violence against persons or property to intimidate or coerce a government, the civilian population, or any segment thereof, in furtherance of political or social objectives."

Both definitions of terrorism share a common theme: the use of force intended to influence or instigate a course of action that furthers a political or social goal.

# How To Help Prevent Terrorist Attacks

This is a message that bears repeating, no matter where you live in the world: Your assistance is needed in preventing terrorist acts.

It's a fact that certain kinds of activities can indicate terrorist plans that are in the works, especially when they occur at or near high profile sites or places where large numbers of people gather—like government buildings, military facilities, utilities, bus or train stations, major public events. If you see or know about suspicious activities, like the ones listed below, please report them immediately to the proper authorities. In the United States, that means your closest Joint Terrorist Task Force, located in an Federal Bureau of Investigation (FBI) field office. In other countries, that means your closest law enforcement/counterterrorism agency.

**Surveillance**: Are you aware of anyone video recording or monitoring activities, taking notes, using cameras, maps, binoculars, etc., near key facilities/events?

**Suspicious Questioning**: Are you aware of anyone attempting to gain information in person, by phone, mail, e-mail, etc., regarding a key facility or people who work there?

**Tests of Security**: Are you aware of any attempts to penetrate or test physical security or procedures at a key facility/event?

**Acquiring Supplies:** Are you aware of anyone attempting to improperly acquire explosives, weapons, ammunition, dangerous chemicals, uniforms, badges, flight manuals, access cards or identification for a key facility/event or to legally obtain items under suspicious circumstances that could be used in a terrorist attack?

**Suspicious Persons**: Are you aware of anyone who does not appear to belong in the workplace, neighborhood, business establishment, or near a key facility/event?

**"Dry Runs"**: Have you observed any behavior that appears to be preparation for a terrorist act, such as mapping out routes, playing out scenarios with other people, monitoring key facilities/events, timing traffic lights or traffic flow, or other suspicious activities?

**Deploying Assets**: Have you observed abandoned vehicles, stockpiling of suspicious materials, or persons being deployed near a key facility/event?

If you answered yes to any of the above if you have observed any suspicious activity that may relate to terrorism again, please contact the Joint Terrorist Task Force or law enforcement/counterterrorism agency closest to you immediately. Your tip could save the lives of innocent people, just like you and yours.

# Chapter 31
# Hurting Yourself

Self-harm, sometimes called self-injury, is when a person purposely hurts his or her own body. There are many types of self-injury, and cutting is one type that you may have heard about. If you are hurting yourself, you can learn to stop. Make sure you talk to an adult you trust, and keep reading to learn more.

## What Are Ways People Hurt Themselves?

Some types of injury leave permanent scars or cause serious health problems, sometimes even death. These are some forms of self-injury:

- Cutting yourself (such as using a razor blade, knife, or other sharp object)

- Punching yourself or punching things (like a wall)

- Burning yourself with cigarettes, matches, or candles

- Pulling out your hair

- Poking objects into body openings

- Breaking your bones or bruising yourself

- Poisoning yourself

About This Chapter: Text in this chapter begins with excerpts from "Cutting And Self-Harm," Office on Women's Health (OWH), U.S. Department of Health and Human Services (HHS), January 7, 2015; Text beginning with the heading "How Common Is Self-Harm?" is excerpted from "Self-Harm And Trauma," U.S. Department of Veterans Affairs (VA), August 13, 2015.

# Who Hurts Themselves?

People from all different kinds of backgrounds hurt themselves. Among teens, girls may be more likely to do it than boys.

People of all ages hurt themselves, too, but self-injury most often starts in the teen years.

People who hurt themselves sometimes have other problems like depression, eating disorders, or drug or alcohol abuse.

# Why Do Some Teens Hurt Themselves?

Some teens who hurt themselves keep their feelings bottled up inside. The physical pain then offers a sense of relief, like the feelings are getting out. Some people who hold back strong emotions begin to feel like they have no emotions, and the injury helps them at least feel something.

Some teens say that when they hurt themselves, they are trying to stop feeling painful emotions, like rage, loneliness, or hopelessness. They may injure to distract themselves from the emotional pain. Or they may be trying to feel some sense of control over what they feel.

**If you are depressed, angry, or having a hard time coping,** talk with an adult you trust. You also can contact a helpline. Remember, you have a right to be safe and happy!

**If you are hurting yourself, please get help.** It is possible to get past the urge to hurt yourself. There are other ways to deal with your feelings. You can talk to your parents, your doctor, or another trusted adult, like a teacher or religious leader. Therapy can help you find healthy ways to handle problems.

# What Are Signs Of Self-Injury In Others?

- Having cuts, bruises, or scars
- Wearing long sleeves or pants even in hot weather
- Making excuses about injuries
- Having sharp objects around for no clear reason

# How Can I Help A Friend Who Is Self-Injuring?

If you think a friend may be hurting herself, try to get your friend to talk to a trusted adult. Your friend may need professional help. A therapist can suggest ways to cope with problems without turning to self-injury. If your friend won't get help, you should talk to an adult. This is too much for you to handle alone.

## What If Someone Pressures Me To Hurt Myself?

If someone pressures you to hurt yourself, think about whether you really want a friend who tries to cause you pain. Try to hang out with other people who don't treat you this way. Try to hang out with people who make you feel good about yourself.

## How Common Is Self-Harm?

The rates of self-harm vary widely, depending on how researchers pose their questions about it. It is estimated that in the general public, 2 percent to 6 percent engage in self-harm at some point in their lives. Among students, the rates are higher, ranging from 13 percent to 35 percent.

Rates of self-harm are also higher among those in treatment for mental health problems. Those in treatment who have a diagnosis of posttraumatic stress disorder (PTSD) are more likely to engage in self-harm than those without PTSD.

## What Are Self-Harmers Like?

Self-harmers, as compared to others, have more frequent and more negative feelings such as fear or worry, depression, and aggressive impulses. Links have also been found between self-harm and feeling numb or feeling as if you're outside your body. Often those who self-harm have low self-esteem, and they do not tend to express their feelings. The research is not clear on whether self-harm is more common in women or men.

Those who self-harm appear to have higher rates of PTSD and other mental health problems. Self-harm is most often related to going through trauma in childhood rather than as an adult. Those who self-harm have high rates of:

- Childhood sexual abuse
- Childhood physical abuse
- Emotional neglect
- Bonds with caregivers that are not stable or secure
- Long separations from caregivers

Those who self-harm very often have a history of childhood sexual abuse. For example, in one group of self-harmers, 93 percent said they had been sexually abused in childhood. Some research has looked at whether certain aspects of childhood sexual abuse increase the risk that survivors will engage in self-harm as adults. The findings show that more severe, more frequent, or longer-lasting sexual abuse is linked to an increased risk of engaging in self-harm in one's adult years.

# Why Do People Engage In Self-Harm?

While many ideas have been offered, the answer to this question may vary from person to person. The reasons that are most often given are "To distract yourself from painful feelings" and "To punish yourself." Research on the reasons for self-harm suggests that people engage in self-harm to:

- Decrease symptoms of feeling numb or as if you are outside your body or yourself

- Reduce stress and tension

- Block upsetting memories and flashbacks

- Show a need for help

- Ensure that you will be safe and protected

- Express and release distress

- Reduce anger

- Punish self

- Hurt self instead of others

# How Is Self-Harm Treated?

Self-harm is a problem that many people are embarrassed or ashamed to discuss. Often, they try to hide their self-harm behaviors. They may hold back from getting mental health or even medical treatment.

Self-harm is often seen with other mental health problems like PTSD or substance abuse. For this reason, it does not tend to be treated separately from the other mental health problems. Some research suggests, though, that adding in a round of therapy focused just on the self-harming behavior may result in less self-harming.

There have not yet been strong studies on using medicine to treat self-harm behaviors. For this reason, experts have not reached agreement on whether medicines should be used to treat self-harm behaviors.

# Chapter 32
# Teen Suicide

## Why Do Teens Try To Kill Themselves?

Most teens interviewed after making a suicide attempt say that they did it because they were trying to escape from a situation that seemed impossible to deal with or to get relief from really bad thoughts or feelings. They didn't want to die as much as they wanted to escape from what was going on. And at that particular moment dying seemed like the only way out.

Some people who end their lives or attempt suicide might be trying to escape feelings of rejection, hurt, or loss. Others might feel angry, ashamed, or guilty about something. Some people may be worried about disappointing friends or family members. And some may feel unwanted, unloved, victimized, or like they're a burden to others.

We all feel overwhelmed by difficult emotions or situations sometimes. But most people get through it or can put their problems in perspective and find a way to carry on with determination and hope. So why does one person try suicide when another person in the same tough situation does not? What makes some people more resilient (better able to deal with life's setbacks and difficulties) than others? What makes a person unable to see another way out of a bad situation besides ending his or her life?

The answer to those questions lies in the fact that most people who commit suicide have depression.

---

About This Chapter: Text in this chapter is excerpted from "Suicide," © 1995–2016. The Nemours Foundation/KidsHealth®. Reprinted with permission.

# Depression

Depression leads people to focus mostly on failures and disappointments, to emphasize the negative side of their situations, and to downplay their own capabilities or worth. Someone with severe depression is unable to see the possibility of a good outcome and may believe they will never be happy or things will never go right for them again.

Depression affects a person's thoughts in such a way that the person doesn't see when a problem can be overcome. It's as if the depression puts a filter on the person's thinking that distorts things. That's why depressed people don't realize that suicide is a permanent solution to a temporary problem in the same way that other people do. A teen with depression may feel like there's no other way out of problems, no other escape from emotional pain, or no other way to communicate a desperate unhappiness.

Sometimes people who feel suicidal may not even realize they are depressed. They're unaware that it is the depression—not the situation—that's influencing them to see things in a "there's no way out," "it will never get better," "there's nothing I can do" kind of way.

When depression lifts because someone gets the proper therapy or treatment, the distorted thinking is cleared. The person can find pleasure, energy, and hope again. But while someone is seriously depressed, suicidal thinking is a real concern.

People with a condition called bipolar disorder are also more at risk for suicide because their condition can cause them to go through times when they are extremely depressed as well as times when they have abnormally high or frantic energy (called mania or manic). Both of these extreme phases of bipolar disorder affect and distort a person's mood, outlook, and judgment. For people with this condition, it can be a challenge to keep problems in perspective and act with good judgment.

# Substance Abuse

Teens with alcohol and drug problems are also more at risk for suicidal thinking and behavior. Alcohol and some drugs have depressive effects on the brain. Misuse of these substances can bring on serious depression. That's especially true for some teens who already have a tendency to depression because of their biology, family history, or other life stressors.

The problem can be made worse because many people who are depressed turn to alcohol or drugs as an escape. But they may not realize that the depressive effects alcohol and drugs have on the brain can actually intensify depression in the long run.

In addition to their depressive effects, alcohol and drugs alter a person's judgment. They interfere with the ability to assess risk, make good choices, and think of solutions to problems. Many suicide attempts occur when someone is under the influence of alcohol or drugs.

This doesn't mean that everyone who is depressed or who has an alcohol or drug problem will try to kill themselves, of course. But these conditions—especially both together—increase a person's risk for suicide.

# Suicide Is Not Always Planned

Sometimes a depressed person plans a suicide in advance. Many times, though, suicide attempts happen impulsively, in a moment of feeling desperately upset. A situation like a breakup, a big fight with a parent, an unintended pregnancy, being outed by someone else, or being victimized in any way can cause someone to feel desperately upset. Often, a situation like this, on top of an existing depression, acts like the final straw.

Some people who attempt suicide mean to die and some aren't completely sure they want to die. For some, a suicide attempt is a way to express deep emotional pain. They can't say how they feel, so, for them, attempting suicide feels like the only way to get their message across. Sadly, many people who really didn't mean to kill themselves end up dead or critically ill.

# Warning Signs

There are often signs that someone may be thinking about or planning a suicide attempt. Here are some of them:

- talking about suicide or death in general

- talking about "going away"

- referring to things they "won't be needing," and giving away possessions

- talking about feeling hopeless or feeling guilty

- pulling away from friends or family and losing the desire to go out

- having no desire to take part in favorite things or activities

- having trouble concentrating or thinking clearly

- experiencing changes in eating or sleeping habits

- engaging in self-destructive behavior (drinking alcohol, taking drugs, or cutting, for example)

# What If This Is You?

If you have been thinking about suicide, get help now. Depression is powerful. You can't wait and hope that your mood might improve. When a person has been feeling down for a long time, it's hard to step back and be objective.

Talk to someone you trust as soon as you can. If you can't talk to a parent, talk to a coach, a relative, a school counselor, a religious leader, or a teacher. Call a suicide crisis line (such as 1-800-SUICIDE) or your local emergency number (911).

These toll-free lines are staffed 24 hours a day, 7 days a week by trained professionals who can help you without ever knowing your name or seeing your face. All calls are confidential— no one you know will find out that you've called. They are there to help you figure out how to work through tough situations.

# What If It's Someone You Know?

It is always a good thing to start a conversation with someone you think may be considering suicide. It allows you to get help for the person, and just talking about it may help the person to feel less alone and more cared about and understood.

Talking things through also may give the person an opportunity to consider other solutions to problems. Most of the time, people who are considering suicide are willing to talk if someone asks them out of concern and care. Because people who are depressed are not as able to see answers as well as others, it can help to have someone work with them in coming up with at least one other way out of a bad situation.

Even if a friend or classmate swears you to secrecy, you must get help as soon as possible— your friend's life could depend on it. Someone who is seriously thinking about suicide may have sunk so deeply into an emotional hole that the person could be unable to recognize that he or she needs help. Tell an adult you trust as soon as possible.

If necessary, you can also call a suicide crisis line (such as 1-800-SUICIDE) or your local emergency number (911). These are confidential resources and the people at any of these places are happy to talk to you to help you figure out what to do.

Sometimes, teens who make a suicide attempt—or who die as a result of suicide—seem to give no clue beforehand. This can leave loved ones feeling not only grief stricken but guilty and wondering if they missed something. It is important for family members and friends of those who die by suicide to know that sometimes there is no warning and they should not blame themselves.

When someone dies by suicide, the people left behind can wrestle with a terrible emotional pain. Teens who have had a recent loss or crisis or who had a family member or classmate who committed suicide may be especially vulnerable to suicidal thinking and behavior themselves.

If you've been close to someone who has attempted or committed suicide, it can help to talk with a therapist or counselor—someone who is trained in dealing with this complex issue. Or, you could join a group for survivors where you can share your feelings and get the support of people who have been in the same situation as you.

# Coping With Problems

Being a teen is not easy. There are many new social, academic, and personal pressures. And for teens who have additional problems to deal with, such as living in violent or abusive environments, life can feel even more difficult.

Some teens worry about sexuality and relationships, wondering if their feelings and attractions are normal, or if they will be loved and accepted. Others struggle with body image and eating problems; trying to reach an impossible ideal leaves them feeling bad about themselves.

Some teens have learning problems or attention problems that make it hard for them to succeed in school. They may feel disappointed in themselves or feel they are a disappointment to others.

These problems can be difficult and draining—and can lead to depression if they go on too long without relief or support. We all struggle with painful problems and events at times. How do people get through it without becoming depressed? Part of it is staying connected to family, friends, school, faith, and other support networks.

People are better able to deal with tough circumstances when they have at least one person who believes in them, wants the best for them, and in whom they can confide. People also cope better when they keep in mind that most problems are temporary and can be overcome.

When struggling with problems, it helps to:

- Tell someone you trust what's going on with you.

- Be around people who are caring and positive.

- Ask someone to help you figure out what to do about a problem you're facing.

- Work with a therapist or counselor if problems are getting you down and depressed—or if you don't have a strong support network or feel you can't cope.

Counselors and therapists can provide emotional support and can help teens build their own coping skills for dealing with problems. It can also help to join a support network for people who are going through the same problems—for example, anorexia and body image issues, living with an alcoholic family member, or sexuality and sexual health concerns. These groups can help provide a caring environment where you can talk through problems with people who share your concerns.

# Chapter 33

# Lesbian, Gay, Bisexual, And Transgender (LGBT) And Violence

Most lesbian, gay, bisexual, transgender, and questioning (LGBTQ) youth are happy and thrive during their adolescent years. Going to a school that creates a safe and supportive learning environment for all students and having caring and accepting parents are especially important. This helps all youth achieve good grades and maintain good mental and physical health. However, some LGBTQ youth are more likely than their heterosexual peers to experience difficulties in their lives and school environments, such as violence.

## Experiences With Violence

Negative attitudes toward lesbian, gay, and bisexual (LGB) people put these youth at increased risk for experiences with violence, compared with other students. Violence can include behaviors such as bullying, teasing, harassment, physical assault, and suicide-related behaviors.

According to data from Youth Risk Behavior Surveys (YRBS) conducted during 2001–2009 in seven states and six large urban school districts, the percentage of LGB students (across the sites) who were threatened or injured with a weapon on school property in the prior year ranged from 12 percent to 28 percent. In addition, across the sites?

- 19 percent to 29 percent of gay and lesbian students and 18 percent to 28 percent of bisexual students experienced dating violence in the prior year.

- 14 percent to 31 percent of gay and lesbian students and 17 percent to 32 percent of bisexual students had been forced to have sexual intercourse at some point in their lives.

About This Chapter: This chapter includes text excerpted from "Lesbian, Gay, Bisexual, And Transgender Health," Centers for Disease Control and Prevention (CDC), November 12, 2014.

LGBTQ youth are also at increased risk for suicidal thoughts and behaviors, suicide attempts, and suicide. A nationally representative study of adolescents in grades 7–12 found that lesbian, gay, and bisexual youth were more than twice as likely to have attempted suicide as their heterosexual peers. More studies are needed to better understand the risks for suicide among transgender youth. However, one study with 55 transgender youth found that about 25 percent reported suicide attempts.

Another survey of more than 7,000 seventh- and eighth-grade students from a large Midwestern county examined the effects of school [social] climate and homophobic bullying on lesbian, gay, bisexual, and questioning (LGBQ) youth and found that:

- LGBQ youth were more likely than heterosexual youth to report high levels of bullying and substance use

- Students who were questioning their sexual orientation reported more bullying, homophobic victimization, unexcused absences from school, drug use, feelings of depression, and suicidal behaviors than either heterosexual or LGB students

- LGB students who did not experience homophobic teasing reported the lowest levels of depression and suicidal feelings of all student groups (heterosexual, LGB, and questioning students)

- All students, regardless of sexual orientation, reported the lowest levels of depression, suicidal feelings, alcohol and marijuana use, and unexcused absences from school when they were:

  - In a positive school climate

  - Not experiencing homophobic teasing

## Effects On Education And Health

Exposure to violence can have negative effects on the education and health of any young person. However, for LGBT youth, a national study of middle and high school students shows that LGBT students (61.1 percent) were more likely than their non-LGBT peers to feel unsafe or uncomfortable as a result of their sexual orientation. According to data from Centers for Disease Control and Prevention's (CDC) YRBS, the percentage of gay, lesbian, and bisexual students (across sites) who did not go to school at least one day during the 30 days before the survey because of safety concerns ranged from 11 percent to 30 percent of gay and lesbian students and 12 percent to 25 percent of bisexual students.

The stresses experienced by LGBT youth also put them at greater risk for depression, substance use, and sexual behaviors that place them at risk for human immunodeficiency virus (HIV) and other sexually transmitted diseases (STDs). For example, HIV infection among young men who have sex with men aged 13–24 years increased by 26 percent over 2008–2011.

## What Schools Can Do

For youth to thrive in their schools and communities, they need to feel socially, emotionally, and physically safe and supported. A positive school climate has been associated with decreased depression, suicidal feelings, substance use, and unexcused school absences among LGBQ students.

Schools can implement clear policies, procedures, and activities designed to promote a healthy environment for all youth. For example, research has shown that in schools with LGB support groups (such as gay-straight alliances), LGB students were less likely to experience threats of violence, miss school because they felt unsafe, or attempt suicide than those students in schools without LGB support groups. Researchers found that LGB students had fewer suicidal thoughts and attempts when schools had gay-straight alliances and policies prohibiting expression of homophobia in place for 3 or more years.

To help promote health and safety among LGBTQ youth, schools can implement the following policies and practices:

- Encourage respect for all students and prohibit bullying, harassment, and violence against all students.

- Identify "safe spaces," such as counselors' offices, designated classrooms, or student organizations, where LGBTQ youth can receive support from administrators, teachers, or other school staff.

- Encourage student-led and student-organized school clubs that promote a safe, welcoming, and accepting school environment (e.g., gay-straight alliances, which are school clubs open to youth of all sexual orientations).

- Ensure that health curricula or educational materials include HIV, other STD, or pregnancy prevention information that is relevant to LGBTQ youth (such as, ensuring that curricula or materials use inclusive language or terminology).

- Encourage school district and school staff to develop and publicize trainings on how to create safe and supportive school environments for all students, regardless of sexual orientation or gender identity, and encourage staff to attend these trainings.

- Facilitate access to community-based providers who have experience providing health services, including HIV/STD testing and counseling, to LGBTQ youth.

- Facilitate access to community-based providers who have experience in providing social and psychological services to LGBTQ youth.

# What Parents Can Do

How parents respond to their LGB teen can have a tremendous impact on their adolescent's current and future mental and physical health. Supportive reactions can help youth cope with the challenges of being an LGBTQ teen. However, some parents react negatively to learning that they may have an LGBTQ daughter or son. In some cases, parents no longer allow their teens to remain in the home. In other situations, stress and conflict at home can cause some youth to run away. As a result, LGB youth are at greater risk for homelessness than their heterosexual peers.

To be supportive, parents should talk openly with their teen about any problems or concerns and be watchful of behaviors that might indicate their child is a victim of bullying or violence—or that their child may be victimizing others. If bullying, violence, or depression is suspected, parents should take immediate action, working with school personnel and other adults in the community.

---

## Ways Parents Can Influence the Health of Their LGB Youth

More research is needed to better understand the associations between parenting and the health of LGB youth. Following are selected research-based steps parents can take to support the health and well-being of their LGB teen:

- **Talk and listen.** Parents who talk with and listen to their teen in a way that invites an open discussion about sexual orientation can help their teen feel loved and supported. Parents should have honest conversations with their teens about sex, and about how to avoid risky behavior and unsafe or high-risk situations.

- **Provide support.** Parents who take time to come to terms with how they feel about their teen's sexual orientation will be more able to respond calmly and use respectful language. Parents should develop common goals with their teen, including being healthy and doing well in school.

- **Stay involved.** Parents who make an effort to know their teen's friends and know what their teen is doing can help their teen stay safe and feel cared about.

- **Be proactive.** Parents can access many organizations and online information resources to learn more about how they can support their LGB teen, other family members, and their teen's friends.

---

# Part Three
Recognizing And Treating The Consequences Of Abuse And Violence

# Chapter 34
# What To Do After A Sexual Assault

## What Is Sexual Assault?

Sexual assault is any type of sexual activity, including rape, that you do not agree to. Also called sexual violence or abuse, sexual assault is never your fault.

## What Is Rape?

Th e Department of Justice (DOJ) defines rape as "The penetration, no matter how slight, of the vagina or anus with any body part or object, or oral penetration by a sex organ of another person, without the consent of the victim." This legal definition is used by the federal government to collect information from local police about rape. The definition of rape may be slightly different in your community.

Rape also can happen when you cannot physically give consent, such as while you were drunk, passed out, or high. Rape can also happen when you cannot legally give consent, such as when you are underage.

## What Does Sexual Assault Include?

Sexual assault can include:

- Any type of sexual contact with someone who cannot consent, such as someone who is underage, has an intellectual disability, or is passed out

About This Chapter: Text beginning with the heading "What Is Sexual Assault?" is excerpted from "Sexual Assault," Office on Women's Health (OWH), May 21, 2015; Text beginning with the heading "Treatment" is excerpted from "Sexual Assault And Abuse And STDs," Centers for Disease Control and Prevention (CDC), June 4, 2015.

- Rape

- Attempted rape

- Sexual coercion

- Sexual contact with a child

- Incest (sexual contact between family members)

- Fondling or unwanted touching above or under clothes

Sexual assault can also be verbal or visual. It is anything that forces a person to join in unwanted sexual contact or attention. Examples can include:

- Voyeurism, or peeping (when someone watches private sexual acts without consent)

- Exhibitionism (when someone exposes himself or herself in public)

- Sexual harassment or threats

- Forcing someone to pose for sexual pictures

# What Do I Do If I've Been Sexually Assaulted?

**If you are in danger or need medical care, call 9-1-1.** If you can, get away from the person who assaulted you and get to a safe place as fast as you can.

If you have been physically assaulted or raped, there are other important steps you can take right away:

- **Save everything that might have the attacker's DNA on it.** As hard as it may be to not wash up, you might wash away important evidence if you do. Don't brush, comb, or clean any part of your body. Don't change clothes, if possible. Don't touch or change anything at the scene of the assault. That way the local police will have physical evidence from the person who assaulted you.

- **Go to your nearest hospital emergency room as soon as possible.** You need to be examined and treated for injuries. You can be given medicine to prevent human immunodeficiency virus (HIV) and other sexually transmitted infections (STIs) and emergency contraception to prevent pregnancy. The National Sexual Assault Hotline at 800-656-HOPE (800-656-4673) can help you find a hospital able to collect evidence of sexual assault. Ask for a sexual assault forensic examiner (SAFE). A doctor or nurse will use a rape kit to collect evidence. This might be fibers, hairs, saliva, semen, or clothing left behind by the attacker. **You do not have to decide whether to press charges while at the hospital.**

If you think you were drugged, talk to the hospital staff about being tested for date rape drugs, such as Rohypnol and Gamma Hydroxybutyrate (GHB), and other drugs.

The hospital staff can also connect you with the local rape crisis center. Staff there can help you make choices about reporting the sexual assault and getting help through counseling and support groups.

- **Reach out for help.** Call a friend or family member you trust, or call a crisis center or hotline. Crisis centers and hotlines have trained volunteers and counselors who can help you find support and resources near you. One hotline is the National Sexual Assault Hotline at 800-656-HOPE (800-656-4673). If you are in the military, you may also call the DoD Safe Helpline at 877-995-5246.

- **Report the sexual assault to the police: Call 911.** If you want to talk to someone first about reporting the assault, you can also call the National Sexual Assault Hotline at 800-656-HOPE (800-656-4673). A counselor can help you understand how to report the crime. Even though these calls are free, they may appear on your phone bill. If you think that the person who sexually assaulted you may check your phone bill, try to call from a friend's phone or a public phone.

- **Write down the details** about the person who sexually assaulted you and what happened.

## Lower Your Risk Of Sexual Assault
- Go to parties or gatherings with friends.
- Look out for your friends, and ask them to look out for you.
- Have a code word with your family and friends.
- Download an app on your phone.
- Avoid drinks in punchbowls or other containers that can be easily "spiked."
- Know your limits when using alcohol or drugs.
- Trust your instincts.
- Be aware of your surroundings.

# Treatment

Compliance with follow-up visits is poor among survivors of sexual assault. As a result, the following routine presumptive treatment after a sexual assault is recommended:

- An empiric antimicrobial regimen for chlamydia, gonorrhea, and trichomonas.

- Emergency contraception. This measure should be considered when the assault could result in pregnancy in the survivor.

- Postexposure hepatitis B vaccination (without hepatitis B immune globulin (HBIG)) if the hepatitis status of the assailant is unknown and the survivor has not been previously vaccinated. If the assailant is known to be HBsAg-positive, unvaccinated survivors should receive both hepatitis B vaccine and HBIG. The vaccine and HBIG, if indicated, should be administered to sexual assault survivors at the time of the initial examination, and follow-up doses of vaccine should be administered 1–2 and 4–6 months after the first dose. Survivors who were previously vaccinated but did not receive postvaccination testing should receive a single vaccine booster dose.

- Human papillomavirus (HPV) vaccination is recommended for female survivors aged 9–26 years and male survivors aged 9–21 years. For methylsulfonylmethane (MSM) with who have not received HPV vaccine or who have been incompletely vaccinated, vaccine can be administered through age 26 years. The vaccine should be administered to sexual assault survivors at the time of the initial examination, and follow-up dose administered at 1–2 months and 6 months after the first dose.

- Recommendations for HIV post-exposure prophylaxis (PEP) are individualized according to risk.

## Recommended Regimens

**Ceftriaxone** 250 mg IM in a single dose

PLUS

**Azithromycin** 1 g orally in a single dose

PLUS

**Metronidazole** 2 g orally in a single dose

OR

**Tinidazole** 2 g orally in a single dose

If alcohol has been recently ingested or emergency contraception is provided, metronidazole or tinidazole can be taken by the sexual assault survivor at home rather than as directly observed therapy to minimize potential side effects and drug interactions. Clinicians should counsel persons regarding the possible benefits and toxicities associated with these treatment regimens; gastrointestinal side effects can occur with this combination. The efficacy of these regimens in preventing infections after sexual assault has not been evaluated. For those requiring alternative treatments, refer to the specific sections in this report relevant to the specific organism.

# Other Management Considerations

At the initial examination and, if indicated, at follow-up examinations, patients should be counseled regarding symptoms of sexually transmitted diseases (STDs) and the need for immediate examination if symptoms occur. Further, they should be instructed to abstain from sexual intercourse until STD prophylactic treatment is completed.

# Follow-Up

After the initial postassault examination, follow-up examinations provide an opportunity to

1. detect new infections acquired during or after the assault

2. complete hepatitis B and HPV vaccinations, if indicated

3. complete counseling and treatment for other STDs; and

4. monitor side effects and adherence to postexposure prophylactic medication, if prescribed.

If initial testing was done, follow-up evaluation should be conducted within 1 week to ensure that results of positive tests can be discussed promptly with the survivor, treatment is provided if not given at the initial visit, and any follow-up for the infection(s) can be arranged. If initial tests are negative and treatment was not provided, examination for STDs can be repeated within 1–2 weeks of the assault; repeat testing detects infectious organisms that might not have reached sufficient concentrations to produce positive test results at the time of initial examination. For survivors who are treated during the initial visit, regardless of whether testing was performed, posttreatment testing should be conducted only if the survivor reports having symptoms. A follow-up examination at 1–2 months should also be considered to reevaluate for development of anogenital warts, especially among sexual assault survivors who received a diagnosis of other STDs. If initial test results were negative and infection in the assailant cannot be ruled out, serologic tests for syphilis can be repeated at 4–6 weeks and 3 months; HIV testing can be repeated at 6 weeks and at 3 and 6 months using methods to identify acute HIV infection.

# Risk For Acquiring HIV Infection

HIV seroconversion has occurred in persons whose only known risk factor was sexual assault or sexual abuse, but the frequency of this occurrence likely is low. In consensual sex, the per-act risk for HIV transmission from vaginal intercourse is 0.1 percent–0.2 percent, and for receptive rectal intercourse, 0.5 percent–3 percent. The per-act risk for HIV transmission from oral sex is substantially lower. Specific circumstances of an assault (e.g., bleeding, which often accompanies trauma) might increase risk for HIV transmission in cases involving vaginal, anal, or oral penetration. Site of exposure to ejaculate, viral load in ejaculate, and the presence of an STD or genital lesions in the assailant or survivor also might increase risk for HIV.

Post-exposure prophylaxis with a 28-day course of zidovudine was associated with an 81 percent reduction in risk for acquiring HIV in a study of healthcare workers who had percutaneous exposures to HIV-infected blood. On the basis of these results and results from animal studies, PEP has been recommended for healthcare workers who have occupational exposures to HIV. These findings have been extrapolated to nonoccupational injection and sexual HIV exposures, including sexual assault. The possibility of HIV exposure from the assault should be assessed at the initial examination; survivors determined to be at risk for HIV should be informed about the possible benefit of non-occupational post-exposure prophylaxis (nPEP) in preventing HIV infection. Initiation of nPEP as soon as possible after the exposure increases the likelihood of prophylactic benefit.

Several factors impact the medical recommendation for nPEP and affect the assault survivor's acceptance of that recommendation, including

1. the likelihood of the assailant having HIV

2. any exposure characteristics that might increase the risk for HIV transmission

3. the time elapsed after the event; and

4. the potential benefits and risks associated with the nPEP

Determination of the assailant's HIV status at the time of the assault examination is usually not possible. Therefore, healthcare providers should assess any available information concerning the

- characteristics and HIV risk behaviors of the assailant(s) (e.g., being an MSM or using injection drugs)

- local epidemiology of HIV/AIDS, and

- exposure characteristics of the assault

When an assailant's HIV status is unknown, determinations regarding risk for HIV transmission to the survivor should be based on

1.  whether vaginal or anal penetration occurred

2.  whether ejaculation occurred on mucous membranes

3.  whether multiple assailants were involved

4.  whether mucosal lesions are present in the assailant or survivor; and

5.  any other characteristics of the assault, survivor, or assailant that might increase risk for HIV transmission

If nPEP is offered, the following information should be discussed with the survivor:

1.  the necessity of early initiation of nPEP to optimize potential benefits (i.e., as soon as possible after and up to 72 hours after the assault)

2.  the importance of close follow-up

3.  the benefit of adherence to recommended dosing; and

4.  potential adverse effects of antiretrovirals

Providers should emphasize that severe adverse effects are rare from nPEP. Clinical management of the survivor should be implemented according to the HIV nPEP guidelines and in collaboration with specialists. However, distress after an assault also might prevent the survivor from accurately weighing exposure risks and benefits of nPEP and from making an informed decision regarding initiating therapy, even when such therapy is considered warranted by the healthcare provider. In this instance, the survivor can be provided a 3–5-day supply of nPEP and scheduled for follow-up at a time that allows for provision of the remaining 23 days of medication (if nPEP has been initiated by the survivor) without interruption in dosing. A follow-up visit also creates opportunity for additional counseling as needed.

Recommendations for postexposure HIV risk assessment of adolescent and adult survivors within 72 hours of sexual assault

*   Assess risk for HIV infection in the assailant, and test that person for HIV whenever possible.

*   Use the algorithm to evaluate the survivor for the need for HIV nPEP.

*   Consult with a specialist in HIV treatment if nPEP is being considered.

*   If the survivor appears to be at risk for acquiring HIV from the assault, discuss nPEP, including benefits and risks.

- If the survivor chooses to start nPEP, provide enough medication to last until the follow-up visit at 3–7 days after initial assessment and assess tolerance to medications.

- If nPEP is started, perform CBC and serum chemistry at baseline.

- Perform an HIV antibody test at original assessment; repeat at 6 weeks, 3 months, and 6 months.

Assistance with nPEP-related decisions can be obtained by calling the National Clinician's Post-Exposure Prophylaxis Hotline (PEP Line) (telephone: 888-448-4911).

# Chapter 35

# Long-Term Consequences Of Child Abuse And Neglect

## Child Abuse And Neglect: Consequences

Child abuse and neglect affect children's health now and later, and costs to our country are significant. Neglect, physical abuse, custodial interference, and sexual abuse are types of child maltreatment that can lead to poor physical and mental health well into adulthood. The physical, psychological, behavioral and economic consequences of child maltreatment are explained below.

> ### Prevalence
> - An estimated 702,000 children were confirmed by child protective services as being victims of abuse and neglect in 2014.
> - At least one in four children have experienced child neglect or abuse (including physical, emotional, and sexual) at some point in their lives, and one in seven children experienced abuse or neglect in the last year.

### Effects: Child Abuse And Neglect Affect Children Now And Later

- improper brain development

- impaired cognitive (learning ability) and socio-emotional (social and emotional) skills

About This Chapter: Text under the heading "Child Abuse And Neglect: Consequences" is excerpted from "Child Abuse And Neglect: Consequences," Centers for Disease Control and Prevention (CDC), March 28, 2016; Text beginning with the heading "Effects Of Maltreatment On Brain Development" is excerpted from "Understanding The Effects Of Maltreatment On Brain Development," Child Welfare Information Gateway, U.S. Department of Health and Human Services (HHS), April 2015.

- lower language development

- blindness, cerebral palsy from head trauma

- higher risk for heart, lung and liver diseases, obesity, cancer, high blood pressure, and high cholesterol

- anxiety

- smoking, alcoholism and drug abuse

## Physical

- In 2014, approximately 1,580 children died from abuse and neglect across the country—a rate of 2.13 deaths per 100,000 children.

- Abuse and neglect during infancy or early childhood can cause regions of the brain to form and function improperly with long-term consequences on cognitive and language abilities, socioemotional development, and mental health. For example, the stress of chronic abuse may cause a "hyperarousal" response in certain areas of the brain, which may result in hyperactivity and sleep disturbances.

- Children may experience severe or fatal head trauma as a result of abuse. Nonfatal consequences of abusive head trauma include varying degrees of visual impairment (e.g., blindness), motor impairment (e.g., cerebral palsy) and cognitive impairments.

- Children who experience abuse and neglect are also at increased risk for adverse health effects and certain chronic diseases as adults, including heart disease, cancer, chronic lung disease, liver disease, obesity, high blood pressure, high cholesterol, and high levels of C-reactive protein.

## Psychological

- In one long-term study, as many as 80 percent of young adults who had been abused met the diagnostic criteria for at least one psychiatric disorder at age 21. These young adults exhibited many problems, including depression, anxiety, eating disorders, and suicide attempts.

- The stress of chronic abuse may result in anxiety and may make victims more vulnerable to problems, such as posttraumatic stress disorder, conduct disorder, and learning, attention, and memory difficulties.

## Behavioral

- Children who experience abuse and neglect are at increased risk for smoking, alcoholism, and drug abuse as adults, as well as engaging in high-risk sexual behaviors.

- Those with a history of child abuse and neglect are 1.5 times more likely to use illicit drugs, especially marijuana, in middle adulthood.

- Studies have found abused and neglected children to be at least 25 percent more likely to experience problems such as delinquency, teen pregnancy, and low academic achievement. Similarly, a longitudinal study found that physically abused children were at greater risk of being arrested as juveniles, being a teen parent, and less likely to graduate high school.

- A National Institute of Justice (NIJ) study indicated that being abused or neglected as a child increased the likelihood of arrest as a juvenile by 59 percent. Abuse and neglect also increased the likelihood of adult criminal behavior by 28 percent and violent crime by 30 percent.

- Child abuse and neglect can have a negative effect on the ability of both men and women to establish and maintain healthy intimate relationships in adulthood.

## Economic

- The total lifetime economic burden resulting from new cases of fatal and nonfatal child abuse and neglect in the United States in 2008 is approximately $124 billion in 2010 dollars. This economic burden rivals the cost of other high profile public health problems, such as stroke and Type 2 diabetes.

- The estimated average lifetime cost per victim of nonfatal child abuse and neglect was $210,012 (in 2010 dollars), including

  - childhood healthcare costs

  - adult medical costs

  - productivity losses

  - child welfare costs

  - criminal justice costs

  - special education costs

The estimated average lifetime cost per death is $1,272,900, including medical costs and productivity losses.

# Effects Of Maltreatment On Brain Development

Just as positive experiences can assist with healthy brain development, children's experiences with child maltreatment or other forms of toxic stress, such as domestic violence or disasters, can negatively affect brain development. This includes changes to the structure and chemical activity of the brain (e.g., decreased size or connectivity in some parts of the brain) and in the emotional and behavioral functioning of the child (e.g., over-sensitivity to stressful situations). For example, healthy brain development includes situations in which babies' babbles, gestures, or cries bring reliable, appropriate reactions from their caregivers. These caregiver-child interactions—sometimes referred to as "serve and return"—strengthen babies' neuronal pathways regarding social interactions and how to get their needs met, both physically and emotionally. If children live in a chaotic or threatening world, one in which their caregivers respond with abuse or chronically provide no response, their brains may become hyperalert for danger or not fully develop. These neuronal pathways that are developed and strengthened under negative conditions prepare children to cope in that negative environment, and their ability to respond to nurturing and kindness may be impaired.

The specific effects of maltreatment may depend on such factors as the age of the child at the time of the maltreatment, whether the maltreatment was a one-time incident or chronic, the identity of the abuser (e.g., parent or other adult), whether the child had a dependable nurturing individual in his or her life, the type and severity of the maltreatment, the intervention, how long the maltreatment lasted, and other individual and environmental characteristics.

# Effects Of Maltreatment On Brain Structure And Activity

Toxic stress, including child maltreatment, can have a variety of negative effects on children's brains:

- **Hippocampus:** Adults who were maltreated may have reduced volume in the hippocampus, which is central to learning and memory. Toxic stress also can reduce the hippocampus's capacity to bring cortisol levels back to normal after a stressful event has occurred.

- **Corpus callosum:** Maltreated children and adolescents tend to have decreased volume in the corpus callosum, which is the largest white matter structure in the brain and is responsible for interhemispheric communication and other processes (e.g., arousal, emotion, higher cognitive abilities).

- **Cerebellum:** Maltreated children and adolescents tend to have decreased volume in the cerebellum, which helps coordinate motor behavior and executive functioning.

- **Prefrontal cortex:** Some studies on adolescents and adults who were severely neglected as children indicate they have a smaller prefrontal cortex, which is critical to behavior, cognition, and emotion regulation, but other studies show no differences. Physically abused children also may have reduced volume in the orbitofrontal cortex, a part of the prefrontal cortex that is central to emotion and social regulation.

- **Amygdala:** Although most studies have found that amygdala volume is not affected by maltreatment, abuse and neglect can cause overactivity in that area of the brain, which helps determine whether a stimulus is threatening and trigger emotional responses.

- **Cortisol levels:** Many maltreated children, both in institutional and family settings, and especially those who experienced severe neglect, tend to have lower than normal morning cortisol levels coupled with flatter release levels throughout the day. (Typically, children have a sharp increase in cortisol in the morning followed by a steady decrease throughout the day.) On the other hand, children in foster care who experienced severe emotional maltreatment had higher than normal morning cortisol levels. These results may be due to the body reacting differently to different stressors. Abnormal cortisol levels can have many negative effects. Lower cortisol levels can lead to decreased energy resources, which could affect learning and socialization; externalizing disorders; and increased vulnerability to autoimmune disorders. Higher cortisol levels could harm cognitive processes, subdue immune and inflammatory reactions, or heighten the risk for affective disorders.

- **Other:** Children who experienced severe neglect early in life while in institutional settings often have decreased electrical activity in their brains, decreased brain metabolism, and poorer connections between areas of the brain that are key to integrating complex information. These children also may continue to have abnormal patterns of adrenaline activity years after being adopted from institutional settings. Additionally, malnutrition, a form of neglect, can impair both brain development (e.g., slowing the growth of neurons, axons, and synapses) and function (e.g., neurotransmitter syntheses, the maintenance of brain tissue).

We also know that some cases of physical abuse can cause immediate direct structural damage to a child's brain. For example, according to the National Center on Shaken Baby Syndrome, shaking a child can destroy brain tissue and tear blood vessels. In the short-term, this can lead to seizures, loss of consciousness, or even death. In the long-term, shaking can damage the fragile brain so that a child develops a range of sensory impairments, as well as cognitive, learning, and behavioral disabilities. Other types of head injuries caused by physical abuse can have similar effects.

# Effects Of Maltreatment On Behavioral, Social, And Emotional Functioning

The changes in brain structure and chemical activity caused by child maltreatment can have a wide variety of effects on children's behavioral, social, and emotional functioning.

**Persistent Fear Response.** Chronic stress or repeated trauma can result in a number of biological reactions, including a persistent fear state. Chronic activation of the neuronal pathways involved in the fear response can create permanent memories that shape the child's perception of and response to the environment. While this adaptation may be necessary for survival in a hostile world, it can become a way of life that is difficult to change, even if the environment improves. Children with a persistent fear response may lose their ability to differentiate between danger and safety, and they may identify a threat in a nonthreatening situation. For example, a child who has been maltreated may associate the fear caused by a specific person or place with similar people or places that pose no threat. This generalized fear response may be the foundation of future anxiety disorders, such as posttraumatic stress disorder (PTSD).

**Hyperarousal.** When children are exposed to chronic, traumatic stress, their brains sensitize the pathways for the fear response and create memories that automatically trigger that response without conscious thought. This is called hyperarousal. These children may be highly sensitive to nonverbal cues, such as eye contact or a touch on the arm, and they may be more likely to misinterpret them. Consumed with a need to monitor nonverbal cues for threats, their brains are less able to interpret and respond to verbal cues, even when they are in an environment typically considered nonthreatening, like a classroom. While these children are often labeled as learning disabled, the reality is that their brains have developed so that they are constantly on alert and are unable to achieve the relative calm necessary for learning.

**Increased Internalizing Symptoms.** Child maltreatment can lead to structural and chemical changes in the areas of the brain involved in emotion and stress regulation. For example, maltreatment can affect connectivity between the amygdala and hippocampus, which can then initiate the development of anxiety and depression by late adolescence. Additionally, early emotional abuse or severe deprivation may permanently alter the brain's ability to use serotonin, a neurotransmitter that helps produce feelings of well-being and emotional stability.

**Diminished Executive Functioning.** Executive functioning generally includes three components: working memory (being able to keep and use information over a short period of time), inhibitory control (filtering thoughts and impulses), and cognitive or mental flexibility (adjusting to changed demands, priorities, or perspectives). The structural and neurochemical damage caused by maltreatment can create deficits in all areas of executive functioning, even at an early age. Executive functioning skills help people achieve academic and career success, bolster social interactions, and assist in everyday activities. The brain alterations caused by a toxic stress response can result in lower academic achievement, intellectual impairment, decreased IQ, and weakened ability to maintain attention.

**Delayed Developmental Milestones.** Although neglect often is thought of as a failure to meet a child's physical needs for food, shelter, and safety, neglect also can be a failure to meet a child's cognitive, emotional, or social needs. For children to master developmental tasks in these areas, they need opportunities and encouragement from their caregivers. If this stimulation is lacking during children's early years, the weak neuronal pathways that developed in expectation of these experiences may wither and die, and the children may not achieve the usual developmental milestones. For example, babies need to experience face-to-face baby talk and hear countless repetitions of sounds in order to build the brain circuitry that will enable them to start making sounds and eventually say words. If babies' sounds are ignored repeatedly when they begin to babble at around 6 months, their language may be delayed. In fact, neglected children often do not show the rapid growth that normally occurs in language development at 18–24 months. These types of delays may extend to all types of normal development for neglected children, including their cognitive-behavioral, socio-emotional, and physical development.

**Weakened Response to Positive Feedback.** Children who have been maltreated may be less responsive to positive stimuli than nonmaltreated children. A study of young adults who had been maltreated found that they rated monetary rewards less positively than their peers and demonstrated a weaker response to reward cues in the basal ganglia areas of the brain responsible for reward processing.

**Complicated Social Interactions.** Toxic stress can alter brain development in ways that make interaction with others more difficult. Children or youth with toxic stress may find it more challenging to navigate social situations and adapt to changing social contexts. They may perceive threats in safe situations more frequently and react accordingly, and they may have more difficulty interacting with others. For example, a maltreated child may misinterpret a peer's neutral facial expression as anger, which may cause the maltreated child to become aggressive or overly defensive toward the peer.

# Chapter 36
# Seeking Mental Health Services

## What Is Therapy?

Therapy isn't just for mental health. You've probably heard people discussing other types of medical therapy, such as physical therapy or chemotherapy. But the word "therapy" is most often used to mean psychotherapy (sometimes called "talk therapy")—in other words, psychological help to deal with stress or problems.

Psychotherapy is a process that's a lot like learning. Through therapy, people learn about themselves. They discover ways to overcome difficulties, develop inner strengths or skills, or make changes in themselves or their situations. Often, it feels good just to have a person to vent to, and other times it's useful to learn different techniques to help deal with stress.

A psychotherapist (therapist, for short) is a person who has been professionally trained to help people deal with stress or other problems. Psychiatrists, psychologists, social workers, counselors, and school psychologists are the titles of some of the licensed professionals who work as therapists. The letters following a therapist's name (for example, MD, PhD, PsyD, EdD, MA, LCSW, LPC) refer to the particular education and degree that therapist has received.

Some therapists specialize in working with a certain age group or on a particular type of problem. Other therapists treat a mix of ages and issues. Some work in hospitals, clinics, or counseling centers. Others work in schools or in psychotherapy offices, often called a "private practice" or "group practice."

---

About This Chapter: Text in this chapter is excerpted from "Going To A Therapist," © 1995–2016. The Nemours Foundation/KidsHealth®. Reprinted with permission.

## What Do Therapists Do?

Most types of therapy include talking and listening, building trust, and receiving support and guidance. Sometimes therapists may recommend books for people to read or work through. They may also suggest keeping a journal. Some people prefer to express themselves using art or drawing. Others feel more comfortable just talking.

When a person talks to a therapist about which situations might be difficult for them or what stresses them out, this helps the therapist assess what is going on. The therapist and client then usually work together to set therapy goals and figure out what will help the person feel better or get back on track.

It might take a few meetings with a therapist before people really feel like they can share personal stuff. It's natural to feel that way. Trust is an essential ingredient in therapy—after all, therapy involves being open and honest about sensitive topics like feelings, ideas, relationships, problems, disappointments, and hopes. A therapist understands that people sometimes take a while to feel comfortable sharing personal information.

Most of the time, a person meets with a therapist one on one, which is known as **individual therapy**. Sometimes, though, a therapist might work with a family (called **family therapy**) or a group of people who all are dealing with similar issues (called **group therapy** or a **support group**). Family therapy gives family members a chance to talk together with a therapist about problems that involve them all. Group therapy and support groups help people give and receive support and learn from each other and their therapist by discussing the issues they have in common.

## What Happens During Therapy?

If you see a therapist, he or she will talk with you about your feelings, thoughts, relationships, and important values. At the beginning, therapy sessions are focused on discussing what you'd like to work on and setting goals. Some of the goals people in therapy may set include things like:

- improving self-esteem and gaining confidence
- figuring out how to make more friends
- feeling less depressed or less anxious
- improving grades at school
- learning to manage anger and frustration
- making healthier choices (for example, about relationships or eating) and ending self-defeating behaviors

During the first visit, your therapist will probably ask you to talk a bit about yourself. Depending on your age, the therapist will also likely meet with a parent or caregiver and ask you to review information regarding confidentiality.

The first meeting can last longer than the usual "therapy hour" and is often called an "intake interview." This helps the therapist understand you better, and gives you a chance to see if you feel comfortable with the therapist. The therapist will probably ask about problems, concerns, and symptoms that you may be having, or the problems that parents or teachers are concerned about.

After one or two sessions, the therapist may talk to you about his or her understanding of what is going on with you, how therapy could help, and what the process will involve. Together, you and your therapist will decide on the goals for therapy and how frequently to meet. This may be once a week, every other week, or once a month.

With a better understanding of your situation, the therapist might teach you new skills or help you to think about a situation in a new way. For example, therapists can help people develop better relationship skills or coping skills, including ways to build confidence, express feelings, or manage anger.

Sticking to the schedule you agree on with your therapist and going to your appointments will ensure you have enough time with your therapist to work out your concerns. If your therapist suggests a schedule that you don't think you'll be able to keep, be up front about it so you can work out an alternative.

## How Private Is It?

Therapists respect the privacy of their clients and they keep things they're told confidential. A therapist won't tell anyone else—including parents—about what a person discusses in his or her sessions unless that person gives permission. The only exception is if therapists believe their clients may harm themselves or others.

If the issue of privacy and confidentiality worries you, be sure to ask your therapist about it during your first meeting. It's important to feel comfortable with your therapist so you can talk openly about your situation.

## Does It Mean I'm Crazy?

No. In fact, many people in your class have probably seen a therapist at some point—just like students often see tutors or coaches for extra help with schoolwork or sports. Getting help in dealing with emotions and stressful situations is as important to your overall health as getting help with a medical problem like asthma or diabetes.

There's nothing wrong with getting help with problems that are hard to solve alone. In fact, it's just the opposite. It takes a lot of courage and maturity to look for solutions to problems instead of ignoring or hiding them and allowing them to become worse. If you think that therapy could help you with a problem, ask an adult you trust—like a parent, school counselor, or doctor—to help you find a therapist.

A few adults still resist the idea of therapy because they don't fully understand it or have outdated ideas about it. A couple of generations ago, people didn't know as much about the mind or the mind-body connection as they do today, and **people** were left to struggle with their problems on their own. It used to be that therapy was only available to those with the most serious mental health problems, but that's no longer the case.

Therapy is helpful to people of all ages and with problems that range from mild to much more serious. Some people still hold on to old beliefs about therapy, such as thinking that teens "will grow out of" their problems. If the adults in your family don't seem open to talking about therapy, mention your concerns to a school counselor, coach, or doctor.

You don't have to hide the fact that you're going to a therapist, but you also don't have to tell anyone if you'd prefer not to. Some people find that talking to a few close friends about their therapy helps them to work out their problems and feel like they're not alone. Other people choose not to tell anyone, especially if they feel that others won't understand. Either way, it's a personal decision.

## What Can A Person Get Out Of Therapy?

What someone gets out of therapy depends on why that person is there. For example, some people go to therapy to solve a specific problem, others want to begin making better choices, and others want to start to heal from a loss or a difficult life situation.

Therapy can help people feel better, be stronger, and make good choices as well as discover more about themselves. Those who work with therapists might learn about motivations that lead them to behave in certain ways or about inner strengths they have. Maybe you'll learn new coping skills, develop more patience, or learn to like yourself better. Maybe you'll find new ways to handle problems that come up or new ways to handle yourself in tough situations.

People who work with therapists often find that they learn a lot about themselves and that therapy can help them grow and mature. Lots of people discover that the tools they learn in therapy when they're young make them feel stronger and better able to deal with whatever life throws at them even as adults. If you are curious about the therapy process, talk to a counselor or therapist to see if you could benefit.

# Chapter 37
# Anxiety Disorders And Depression

## Anxiety Disorders

Occasional anxiety is a normal part of life. You might feel anxious when faced with a problem at work, before taking a test, or making an important decision. But anxiety disorders involve more than temporary worry or fear. For a person with an anxiety disorder, the anxiety does not go away and can get worse over time. The feelings can interfere with daily activities such as job performance, school work, and relationships. There are several different types of anxiety disorders. Examples include generalized anxiety disorder, panic disorder, and social anxiety disorder.

## Signs And Symptoms
### Generalized Anxiety Disorder

People with generalized anxiety disorder display excessive anxiety or worry for months and face several anxiety-related symptoms.

Generalized anxiety disorder symptoms include:

- Restlessness or feeling wound-up or on edge

- Being easily fatigued

- Difficulty concentrating or having their minds go blank

About This Chapter: Text under the heading "Anxiety Disorders" is excerpted from "Anxiety Disorders," National Institute of Mental Health (NIMH), March 2016; Text beginning with the heading "Depression" is excerpted from "Depression And College Students," National Institute of Mental Health (NIMH), November 11, 2015.

- Irritability

- Muscle tension

- Difficulty controlling the worry

- Sleep problems (difficulty falling or staying asleep or restless, unsatisfying sleep)

## Panic Disorder

People with panic disorder have recurrent unexpected panic attacks, which are sudden periods of intense fear that may include palpitations, pounding heart, or accelerated heart rate; sweating; trembling or shaking; sensations of shortness of breath, smothering, or choking; and feeling of impending doom.

Panic disorder symptoms include:

- Sudden and repeated attacks of intense fear

- Feelings of being out of control during a panic attack

- Intense worries about when the next attack will happen

- Fear or avoidance of places where panic attacks have occurred in the past

## Social Anxiety Disorder

People with social anxiety disorder (sometimes called "social phobia") have a marked fear of social or performance situations in which they expect to feel embarrassed, judged, rejected, or fearful of offending others.

Social anxiety disorder symptoms include:

- Feeling highly anxious about being with other people and having a hard time talking to them

- Feeling very self-conscious in front of other people and worried about feeling humiliated, embarrassed, or rejected, or fearful of offending others

- Being very afraid that other people will judge them

- Worrying for days or weeks before an event where other people will be

- Staying away from places where there are other people

- Having a hard time making friends and keeping friends

- Blushing, sweating, or trembling around other people

- Feeling nauseous or sick to your stomach when other people are around

Evaluation for an anxiety disorder often begins with a visit to a primary care provider. Some physical health conditions, such as an overactive thyroid or low blood sugar, as well as taking certain medications, can imitate or worsen an anxiety disorder. A thorough mental health evaluation is also helpful, because anxiety disorders often co-exist with other related conditions, such as depression or obsessive-compulsive disorder.

# Risk Factors

Researchers are finding that genetic and environmental factors, frequently in interaction with one another, are risk factors for anxiety disorders. Specific factors include:

- Shyness, or behavioral inhibition, in childhood

- Being female

- Having few economic resources

- Being divorced or widowed

- Exposure to stressful life events in childhood and adulthood

- Anxiety disorders in close biological relatives

- Parental history of mental disorders

- Elevated afternoon cortisol levels in the saliva (specifically for social anxiety disorder)

# Treatments And Therapies

Anxiety disorders are generally treated with psychotherapy, medication, or both.

## Psychotherapy

Psychotherapy or "talk therapy" can help people with anxiety disorders. To be effective, psychotherapy must be directed at the person's specific anxieties and tailored to his or her needs. A typical "side effect" of psychotherapy is temporary discomfort involved with thinking about confronting feared situations.

### Cognitive Behavioral Therapy (CBT)

CBT is a type of psychotherapy that can help people with anxiety disorders. It teaches a person different ways of thinking, behaving, and reacting to anxiety-producing and fearful situations. CBT can also help people learn and practice social skills, which is vital for treating social anxiety disorder.

Two specific stand-alone components of CBT used to treat social anxiety disorder are **cognitive therapy** and **exposure therapy**. Cognitive therapy focuses on identifying, challenging, and then neutralizing unhelpful thoughts underlying anxiety disorders.

Exposure therapy focuses on confronting the fears underlying an anxiety disorder in order to help people engage in activities they have been avoiding. Exposure therapy is used along with relaxation exercises and/or imagery. One study, called a meta-analysis because it pulls together all of the previous studies and calculates the statistical magnitude of the combined effects, found that cognitive therapy was superior to exposure therapy for treating social anxiety disorder.

CBT may be conducted individually or with a group of people who have similar problems. Group therapy is particularly effective for social anxiety disorder. Often "homework" is assigned for participants to complete between sessions.

## Self-Help Or Support Groups

Some people with anxiety disorders might benefit from joining a self-help or support group and sharing their problems and achievements with others. Internet chat rooms might also be useful, but any advice received over the Internet should be used with caution, as Internet acquaintances have usually never seen each other and false identities are common. Talking with a trusted friend or member of the clergy can also provide support, but it is not necessarily a sufficient alternative to care from an expert clinician.

## Stress-Management Techniques

Stress management techniques and meditation can help people with anxiety disorders calm themselves and may enhance the effects of therapy. While there is evidence that aerobic exercise has a calming effect, the quality of the studies is not strong enough to support its use as treatment. Since caffeine, certain illicit drugs, and even some over-the-counter cold medications can aggravate the symptoms of anxiety disorders, avoiding them should be considered. Check with your physician or pharmacist before taking any additional medications.

The family can be important in the recovery of a person with an anxiety disorder. Ideally, the family should be supportive but not help perpetuate their loved one's symptoms.

## Medication

Medication does not cure anxiety disorders but often relieves symptoms. Medication can only be prescribed by a medical doctor (such as a psychiatrist or a primary care provider), but a few states allow psychologists to prescribe psychiatric medications.

Medications are sometimes used as the initial treatment of an anxiety disorder, or are used only if there is insufficient response to a course of psychotherapy. In research studies, it is common for patients treated with a combination of psychotherapy and medication to have better outcomes than those treated with only one or the other.

The most common classes of medications used to combat anxiety disorders are antidepressants, anti-anxiety drugs, and beta blockers. Be aware that some medications are effective only if they are taken regularly and that symptoms may recur if the medication is stopped.

### Antidepressants

Antidepressants are used to treat depression, but they also are helpful for treating anxiety disorders. They take several weeks to start working and may cause side effects such as headache, nausea, or difficulty sleeping. The side effects are usually not a problem for most people, especially if the dose starts off low and is increased slowly over time.

### Anti-Anxiety Medications

Anti-anxiety medications help reduce the symptoms of anxiety, panic attacks, or extreme fear and worry. The most common anti-anxiety medications are called benzodiazepines. Benzodiazepines are first-line treatments for generalized anxiety disorder. With panic disorder or social phobia (social anxiety disorder), benzodiazepines are usually second-line treatments, behind antidepressants.

### Beta Blockers

Beta blockers, such as propranolol and atenolol, are also helpful in the treatment of the physical symptoms of anxiety, especially social anxiety. Physicians prescribe them to control rapid heartbeat, shaking, trembling, and blushing in anxious situations.

Choosing the right medication, medication dose, and treatment plan should be based on a person's needs and medical situation, and done under an expert's care. Only an expert clinician can help you decide whether the medication's ability to help is worth the risk of a side effect. Your doctor may try several medicines before finding the right one.

You and your doctor should discuss:

- How well medications are working or might work to improve your symptoms

- Benefits and side effects of each medication

- Risk for serious side effects based on your medical history

- The likelihood of the medications requiring lifestyle changes

- Costs of each medication

- Other alternative therapies, medications, vitamins, and supplements you are taking and how these may affect your treatment

- How the medication should be stopped. Some drugs can't be stopped abruptly but must be tapered off slowly under a doctor's supervision.

# Depression

Depression is a medical illness with many symptoms, including physical ones. Sadness is only a small part of depression. Some people with depression may not feel sadness at all, but be more irritable, or just lose interest in things they usually like to do. Depression interferes with your daily life and normal function. Don't ignore or try to hide the symptoms. It is not a character flaw, and you can't will it away.

## Are There Different Types Of Depression?

Yes. The most common depressive disorders include major depression (a discrete episode, clearly different from a person's usual feeling and functioning), persistent depressive disorder (a chronic, low-grade depression that can get better or worse over time), and psychotic depression (the most severe, with delusions or hallucinations). Some people are vulnerable to depression in the winter ("seasonal affective disorder"), and some women report depression in the week or two prior to their menstrual period ("premenstrual dysphoric disorder").

## What Are The Signs And Symptoms Of Depression?

If you have been experiencing any of the following signs and symptoms nearly every day for at least 2 weeks, you may have major (sometimes called "clinical") depression:

- Persistent sad, anxious, or "empty" mood

- Feelings of hopelessness, pessimism

- Feelings of guilt, worthlessness, helplessness

- Loss of interest or pleasure in hobbies and activities

- Decreased energy, fatigue, being "slowed down"

- Difficulty concentrating, remembering, making decisions

- Difficulty sleeping, early-morning awakening, or oversleeping

- Appetite and/or unwanted weight changes

- Thoughts of death or suicide; suicide attempts

- Restlessness, irritability

- Persistent physical symptoms, such as muscle pain or headaches

# What Are "Co-Occurring" Disorders?

Depression can occur at the same time as other health problems, such as anxiety, an eating disorder, or substance abuse. It can also co-occur with other medical conditions, such as diabetes or thyroid imbalance. Certain medications—for example, those for the treatment of severe acne—may cause side effects that contribute to depression; although some women are very sensitive to hormonal changes, modern birth control pills are not associated with depression for most users.

# If I Think I May Have Depression, Where Can I Get Help?

If you have symptoms of depression that are getting in the way of your ability to function with your studies and your social life, ask for help. Depression can get better with care and treatment. Don't wait for depression to go away by itself or think you can manage it all on your own, and don't ignore how you're feeling just because you think you can "explain" it. As a college student, you're busy—but you need to make time to get help. If you don't ask for help, depression may get worse and contribute to other health problems, while robbing you of the academic and social enjoyment and success that brought you to college in the first place. It can also lead to "self-medication" with high-risk behaviors with their own serious consequences, such as binge drinking and other substance abuse and having unsafe sex.

Most colleges provide mental health services through counseling centers, student health centers, or both. Check out your college website for information. If you think you might have depression, start by making an appointment with a doctor or healthcare provider for a checkup. This can be a doctor or healthcare provider at your college's student health services center, a doctor who is off-campus in your college town, or a doctor in your hometown. Your doctor can make sure that you do not have another health problem that is causing your depression.

If your doctor finds that you do not have another health problem, he or she can discuss treatment options or refer you to a mental health professional, such as a psychiatrist, counselor, or psychologist. A mental health professional can give you a thorough evaluation and also treat your depression.

If you have thoughts of wishing you were dead or of suicide, call a helpline, such as 1-800-273-TALK (1-800-273-8255), for free 24-hour help, call campus security or 911, or go to the nearest emergency room.

# How Is Depression Treated?

Effective treatments for depression include talk therapy (also called psychotherapy), personalized for your situation, or a combination of talk therapy and medication. Early treatment is best.

# What Is Talk Therapy?

A therapist, such as a psychiatrist, a psychologist, a social worker, or counselor, can help you understand and manage your moods and feelings. You can talk out your emotions to someone who understands and supports you. You can also learn how to stop thinking negatively and start to look at the positives in life. This will help you build confidence and feel better about yourself as you begin to work with your therapist to find solutions to problems that may have seemed insurmountable when you were feeling depressed and maybe even hopeless. Research has shown that certain types of talk therapy or psychotherapy can help young adults deal with depression.

These include:

- **Cognitive behavioral therapy**, or CBT, which focuses on thoughts, behaviors, and feelings related to depression

- **Interpersonal psychotherapy**, or IPT, which focuses on working on relationships

- **Dialectical behavior therapy**, or DBT, which is especially useful when depression is accompanied by self-destructive or self-harming behavior

All therapies can be adapted to each person's issues, for example, if depression is associated with an anxiety or eating disorder. Your college counseling center may offer both individual and group counseling. Many also offer workshops and outreach programs to support you.

# What Medications Treat Depression?

If your doctor thinks you need medication to help your depression, he or she may prescribe an antidepressant. There are a number of antidepressants that have been widely studied and proven to help. If your doctor recommends medication, it is important to see your doctor regularly and tell him or her about any side effects and how you are feeling, especially if you start feeling worse or have thoughts of hurting yourself. Although the doctor will attempt to "match" the best medication for your depression, sometimes it takes a little "trial and error" to find the best choice. If you or a close family member has done well on a particular medication in the past, that can be a good predictor of success again.

Always follow the directions of the doctor or healthcare provider when taking medication. You will need to take one or more regular doses of an antidepressant every day, and it may not take full effect for a few weeks. To avoid having depression return, most people continue taking medication for some months after they are feeling better. If your depression is long-lasting or comes back repeatedly, you may need to take antidepressants longer.

Although all antidepressants can cause side effects, some are more likely to cause certain side effects than others. Tell your doctor if you are often "sensitive" to medication; starting with a low dose and increasing it slowly to a full therapeutic level is the best way to minimize adverse effects. You may need to try more than one antidepressant medicine before finding the one that improves your symptoms without causing side effects that are difficult to live with.

# Chapter 38
# Posttraumatic Stress Disorder

## What Is Posttraumatic Stress Disorder (PTSD)?

Posttraumatic stress disorder (PTSD) is a disorder that develops in some people who have experienced a shocking, scary, or dangerous event.

It is natural to feel afraid during and after a traumatic situation. Fear triggers many split-second changes in the body to help defend against danger or to avoid it. This "fight-or-flight" response is a typical reaction meant to protect a person from harm. Nearly everyone will experience a range of reactions after trauma, yet most people recover from initial symptoms naturally. Those who continue to experience problems may be diagnosed with PTSD. People who have PTSD may feel stressed or frightened even when they are not in danger.

## What Events Cause PTSD In Children?

Any life threatening event or event that threatens physical harm can cause PTSD. These events may include:

- sexual abuse or violence (does not require threat of harm)

- physical abuse

- natural or man-made disasters, such as fires, hurricanes, or floods

About This Chapter: Text under the heading "What Is Posttraumatic Stress Disorder (PTSD)?" is excerpted from "Posttraumatic Stress Disorder," National Institute of Mental Health (NIMH), February 2016; Text beginning with the heading "What Events Cause PTSD In Children?" is excerpted from "PTSD In Children And Adolescents," U.S. Department of Veterans Affairs (VA), February 23, 2016.

- violent crimes such as kidnapping or school shootings

- motor vehicle accidents such as automobile and plane crashes

PTSD can also occur after witnessing violence. These events may include exposure to:

- community violence

- domestic violence

- war

Finally, in some cases learning about these events happening to someone close to you can cause PTSD.

# How Many Children And Adolescents Experience Traumatic Events?

In 2011, child protective services in the United States received 3.4 million referrals, representing 6.2 million children. Of those cases referred, about 19 percent were substantiated and occurred in the following frequencies.

- More than 75 percent (78.5%) suffered neglect

- More than 15 percent (17.6%) suffered physical abuse.

- Less than 10 percent (9.1%) suffered sexual abuse.

In older children there have been several national studies. The National Survey of Children's Exposure to Violence reports on 1 year and lifetime prevalence of childhood victimization in a nationally representative sample of 4549 children aged 0–17.2 More than half (60.6%) of the sample experienced or witnessed victimization in the past year. Specifically in the past year:

- almost half (46.3%) experienced physical assault

- 1 in 10 (10.2%) experienced child maltreatment

- fewer than 1 in 10 (6.1%) had experienced sexual victimization

- more than 1 in 4 (25.3%) had witnessed domestic or community

As children age there is more opportunity for exposure, thus lifetime exposure was one third to one half higher than past year exposure. As an example, among 14–17 year old girls, 18.7 have experienced a completed or attempted sexual assault in their lifetime and more than a third had witnessed parental assault.

A second national study asked 4,023 adolescents aged 12–17 if they had ever experienced sexual or physical assault or witnessed violence. Almost half (47%) had experienced one of these types of traumas. Specifically in their lifetime:

- 8 percent experienced sexual assault

- 22 percent experienced physical assault

- 39 percent witnessed violence

## How Many Adolescents Develop PTSD?

The National Comorbidity Survey Replication—Adolescent Supplement is a nationally representative sample of over 10,000 adolescents aged 13–18. Results indicate that 5 percent of adolescents have met criteria for PTSD in their lifetime. Prevalence is higher for girls than boys (8.0% vs. 2.3%) and increase with age. Current rates (in the past month) are 3.9 percent overall.

## What Are The Risk Factors For PTSD?

Both the type of event and the intensity of exposure impact the degree to which an event results in PTSD. For example, in one study of a fatal sniper attack that occurred at an elementary school proximity to the shooting was directly related to the percentage of children who developed PTSD. Of those children who directly witnessed the shooting on the playground, 77 percent had moderate to severe PTSD symptoms, whereas 67 percent of those in the school building at the time and only 26 percent of the children who had gone home for the day had moderate or severe symptoms.

In addition to exposure variables, other risk factors include:

- female gender

- previous trauma exposure

- preexisting psychiatric disorders

- parental psychopathology

- low social support

Parents have been shown to have protective factors (practice parameters). Both parental support and lower levels of parental PTSD have been found to predict lower levels of PTSD in children.

# What Does PTSD Look Like In Children?

As in adults, PTSD in children and adolescence requires the presence of re-experiencing, avoidance and numbing, and arousal symptoms. However, researchers and clinicians are beginning to recognize that PTSD may not present itself in children the same way it does in adults. Criteria for PTSD include age-specific features for some symptoms.

## Adolescents And Teens

PTSD in adolescents may begin to more closely resemble PTSD in adults. However, there are a few features that have been shown to differ. Children may engage in traumatic play following a trauma. Adolescents are more likely to engage in traumatic reenactment, in which they incorporate aspects of the trauma into their daily lives.

Posttraumatic play is different from reenactment in that posttraumatic play is a literal representation of the trauma, involves compulsively repeating some aspect of the trauma, and does not tend to relieve anxiety. An example of posttraumatic play is an increase in shooting games after exposure to a school shooting. Posttraumatic reenactment, on the other hand, is more flexible and involves behaviorally recreating aspects of the trauma (e.g., carrying a weapon after exposure to violence).

In addition, adolescents are more likely than younger children or adults to exhibit impulsive and aggressive behaviors.

# Besides PTSD, What Are The Other Effects Of Trauma On Children?

Besides PTSD, children and adolescents who have experienced traumatic events often exhibit other types of problems.

Sexually abused children often have problems with fear, anxiety, depression, anger and hostility, aggression, sexually inappropriate behavior, self-destructive behavior, feelings of isolation and stigma, poor self-esteem, difficulty in trusting others, substance abuse, and sexual maladjustment.

These problems are often seen in children and adolescents who have experienced other types of traumas as well. Children who have experienced traumas also often have relationship problems with peers and family members, problems with acting out, and problems with school performance.

Along with associated symptoms, there are a number of psychiatric disorders that are commonly found in children and adolescents who have been traumatized. One commonly co-occurring disorder is major depression. Other disorders include substance abuse; anxiety disorders such as separation anxiety, panic disorder, and generalized anxiety disorder; and externalizing disorders such as attention deficit hyperactivity disorder (ADHD), oppositional defiant disorder, and conduct disorder.

# How Is PTSD Treated In Children And Adolescents?

Although some children show a natural remission in PTSD symptoms over a period of a few months, a significant number of children continue to exhibit symptoms for years if untreated. Trauma Focused (TF) psychotherapies have the most empirical support for children and adolescents.

## Cognitive-Behavioral Therapy (CBT)

Research studies show that CBT is the most effective approach for treating children. The treatment with the best empirical evidence is Trauma-Focused CBT (TF-CBT). TF-CBT generally includes the child directly discussing the traumatic event (exposure), anxiety management techniques such as relaxation and assertiveness training, and correction of inaccurate or distorted trauma related thoughts.

Although there is some controversy regarding exposing children to the events that scare them, exposure-based treatments seem to be most relevant when memories or reminders of the trauma distress the child. Children can be exposed gradually and taught relaxation so that they can learn to relax while recalling their experiences. Through this procedure, they learn that they do not have to be afraid of their memories.

CBT also involves challenging children's false beliefs such as, "the world is totally unsafe." The majority of studies have found that it is safe and effective to use CBT for children with PTSD.

CBT is often accompanied by psycho-education and parental involvement. Psycho-education is education about PTSD symptoms and their effects. It is as important for parents and caregivers to understand the effects of PTSD as it is for children. Research shows that the better parents cope with the trauma, and the more they support their children, the better their children will function. Therefore, it is important for parents to seek treatment for themselves in order to develop the necessary coping skills that will help their children.

## Psychological First Aid

Psychological First Aid has been used for school-aged children and adolescents exposed to disasters and community violence and can be used in schools and traditional settings. Psychological First Aid involves providing comfort and support, normalizing the children's reactions, helping caregivers deal with changes in the child's emotions and behavior, teaching calming and problem-solving skills, and referring the most symptomatic children for additional treatment.

## Eye Movement Desensitization And Reprocessing (EMDR)

Another therapy, EMDR, combines cognitive therapy with directed eye movements. While EMDR has been shown to be effective in treating adults, research with children is not as strong. Studies indicate that it is the cognitive component rather than the eye movements that accounts for the change.

## Medications

Selective serotonin reuptake inhibitors (SSRI) are approved for use in adults with PTSD. SSRIs are approved for use in children and adolescents with depression and obsessive-compulsive disorder (OCD). Preliminary evidence suggests SSRIs may be effective in treating PTSD; however, there may also be risks such as irritability, poor sleep, and inattention. At this time, there is insufficient evidence to support the use of SSRIs.

## Specialized Interventions

Specialized interventions may be necessary for children exhibiting particularly problematic symptoms or behaviors, such as inappropriate sexual behaviors, extreme behavioral problems, or substance abuse.

# Chapter 39

# Dissociative Disorders

Dissociation is a psychological state that involves feeling disconnected from reality. A dissociative disorder is a mental health condition in which the affected person experiences a disconnection from their thoughts, feelings, memories, perceptions, consciousness, or identity.

For many people, dissociation is used as a defense mechanism to block out the memory of extremely stressful or traumatic life experiences, particularly from childhood. Dissociative disorders are often found in individuals who were exposed to physical, emotional, or sexual abuse as children, for instance, and in those who endured such traumatic events as natural disasters, wars, accidents, violent crimes, or the tragic loss of a loved one. Dissociative disorders often manifest themselves during stressful situations in adulthood, which can make it difficult for people affected to deal with the challenges of everyday life.

Research suggests that around 2 to 3 percent of people are affected by dissociative disorders. Some of the common symptoms include episodes of memory or sensory loss, feelings of emotional detachment, or a sense of watching oneself from the outside. Dissociative disorders often coincide with other mental health issues, such as mood swings, attention deficits, drug and alcohol dependence, anxiety, panic attacks, and suicidal tendencies.

According to the *American Psychiatric Association's Diagnostic and Statistical Manual*, dissociative disorders take three main forms: depersonalization/derealization disorder; dissociative amnesia; and dissociative identity disorder.

# Depersonalization/Derealization Disorder

Depersonalization is a profound sense of detachment or alienation from one's own body, mind, or identity. People with depersonalization disorder may experience an "out of body" sensation, or feel as if they are looking at their own life from an external perspective, like watching a movie. Some people affected by this condition may not recognize their own face in a mirror.

Derealization is the sense that the world does not seem real. People with derealization disorder may report that their surroundings appear hazy, foggy, phony, or far away. Familiar places may seem unfamiliar, and close friends may seem like strangers. In some cases, situations take on a dreamlike quality, and the affected person may feel disoriented and have difficulty determining what is real and what is not.

# Dissociative Amnesia

Dissociative amnesia is the inability to remember people, events, or personal information. This memory loss is too substantial to be considered normal forgetfulness, and it is not related to aging, disease, or a head injury. In most cases, people with dissociative amnesia forget a traumatic incident or an extremely stressful period of time. They may also experience smaller lapses in which they forget the content of a conversation or a talent or skill that they have learned.

Dissociative amnesia may be localized, selective, or generalized. In localized amnesia, the memory lapse is concerned with a particular event or span of time. In selective amnesia, the affected person forgets certain parts of a traumatic incident but may remember others.

In generalized amnesia, the affected person is unable to remember anything about their own identity or life history. In rare cases dissociative amnesia may take the form of fugue, in which a person travels for hours or days without a sense of their own identity, then suddenly regains awareness and wonders how they got there.

# Dissociative Identity Disorder

Dissociative identity disorder, formerly known as multiple personality disorder, is characterized by a deep uncertainty or confusion about one's identity. People affected by this disorder may feel the presence of other people or alternate identities (known as "alters") within themselves.

Each of these alters may have their own name, history, voice, mannerisms, and worldview.

A child who has suffered a severe psychological trauma is more likely to develop a dissociative identity disorder. Since the child's mind lacks the coping mechanisms to process the stressful experience, the still-developing personality may find it easier to dissociate and pretend that it was happening to someone else.

# Treatment For Dissociative Disorders

Before diagnosing a dissociative disorder, a doctor may perform tests to rule out physical conditions that may cause similar symptoms, such as a head injury, brain tumor, sleep deprivation, or drug addiction. If no physical cause is found, the patient may be referred to a mental health professional for further evaluation. The mental health specialist will likely inquire about childhood trauma and screen the patient for trauma-related conditions, such as anxiety, depression, posttraumatic stress disorder, and substance abuse. Although there is no medication to treat dissociation, antidepressants and anti-anxiety drugs may provide some relief from the symptoms of associated conditions.

Psychiatrists often treat dissociative disorders with counseling designed to help the patient cope with the underlying trauma. They view dissociation as a normal defense mechanism that the brain may use to adapt to a difficult situation in early life. Dissociation only becomes dysfunctional when it persists into adulthood and governs an individual's response to everyday challenges. In these cases, the patient may benefit from a course of psychotherapy to help them understand and process the traumatic event.

Eye movement desensitization and reprocessing (EMDR) is another technique that can help alleviate symptoms related to psychological trauma. In EMDR, the patient makes side-to-side eye motions, usually by following the movement of the therapist's finger, while recalling the traumatic incident. Although doctors are not sure how EMDR works, it appears to help the brain process distressing memories so that they have less impact on the patient's daily life.

## References

1. "Dissociative Disorders," National Alliance on Mental Illness, n.d.

2. "Dissociative Disorders," NHS Choices, Gov.UK, 2014.

3. "Dissociation FAQs," International Society for the Study of Trauma and Dissociation, 2014.

# Part Four
## Prevention, Staying Safe, And Your Legal Rights As A Victim

# Chapter 40

# How Can Domestic Violence And Abuse Be Prevented And Treated?

## Prevent Domestic Violence In Your Community

**There are numerous ways to enhance prevention efforts in your community. A key strategy in preventing domestic violence, often called intimate partner violence, is promoting respectful, nonviolent relationships.**

The Centers for Disease Control and Prevention (CDC) is committed to ensuring that all Americans, especially those at risk for intimate partner violence (IPV), live to their fullest potential. The goal is to stop IPV before it begins. Disrupting the developmental pathways toward partner violence and teaching skills that promote respectful, nonviolent relationships through individual, relationship, community, and societal level change are key strategies. Creating protective environments where people work, live, and play and strengthening economic supports for families to make violence less likely are also important.

## What Is Intimate Partner Violence?

Intimate partner violence includes physical violence, sexual violence, threats of physical or sexual violence, stalking, and emotional or psychological abuse by a current or former intimate partner. This type of violence can occur among heterosexual or same-sex couples and does not require sexual intimacy. It exists along a continuum from a single episode of violence to severe episodes over a period of years.

---

About This Chapter: Text beginning with the heading "Prevent Domestic Violence In Your Community" is excerpted from "Prevent Domestic Violence In Your Community," Centers for Disease Control and Prevention (CDC), October 3, 2016; Text under the heading "Testing New And Innovative Prevention Strategies" is excerpted from "Understanding And Preventing Violence," Centers for Disease Control and Prevention (CDC), 2013. Reviewed November 2016; Text beginning with the heading "Help Others Be Violence-Free" is excerpted from "Preventing Youth Violence: Opportunities For Action," Centers for Disease Control and Prevention (CDC), June 2014.

Twenty-seven percent of women and nearly 12 percent of men in the United States have experienced intimate partner violence in the form of physical violence, contact sexual violence, or stalking by an intimate partner and that the violence in that relationship resulted in at least one negative impact.

The key to violence prevention is keeping it from happening before it begins.

# Why Is Intimate Partner Violence A Public Health Problem?

Data from CDC's National Intimate Partner and Sexual Violence Survey (NISVS) indicate:

- Severe physical violence was experienced by 22 percent of women and 14 percent of men. This includes being hit with something hard, being kicked or beaten, or being burned.

- Nine percent of women and 1 percent of men experienced attempted or completed rape by an intimate partner during their lifetime.

- Nine percent of women and 3 percent of men were stalked by an intimate partner during their lifetime.

- Among victims of contact sexual violence, physical violence, or stalking by an intimate partner, 71 percent of women and 58 percent of men first experienced these types of violence before the age of 25.

- Twenty-seven percent of women and nearly 12 percent of men in the United States have experienced contact sexual violence, physical violence, or stalking by an intimate partner and reported that the violence in that relationship impacted them in some way (e.g., made them feel fearful or concerned for their safety, resulted in an injury or need for services, or they lost days from work or school). Contact sexual violence includes rape, being made to penetrate, sexual coercion, and unwanted sexual contact.

# What We Know And Don't Know

All forms of IPV are preventable. The key to violence prevention is keeping it from happening before it begins. We know that strategies that promote healthy behaviors in relationships are important. Programs that teach young people skills (e.g., communication and problem solving) can prevent violence. These programs can stop violence in dating relationships before it occurs.

However, more knowledge about strategies that prevent IPV is needed. CDC researchers are working to better understand the developmental pathways and social circumstances that lead to this type of violence.

# Testing New And Innovative Prevention Strategies
## Preventing Abusive Head Trauma

A leading cause of death from child maltreatment is abusive head trauma, but little is known about how to effectively prevent it. DVP is supporting evaluations of two promising state-wide approaches. Researchers at Pennsylvania State University are examining a program in 16 counties that educates parents of all newborns before leaving the hospital about violent infant shaking and the feasibility of booster sessions delivered to parents during well-baby healthcare appointments. The second study, being conducted by researchers at the University of North Carolina at Chapel Hill, is an evaluation of the *Period of Purple Crying* program, which educates parents of all newborns leaving the hospital and at the first well-baby visit about normal infant crying patterns, how to respond to crying, and the dangers of shaking. The *Period of Purple Crying* program also includes a media campaign to reinforce program messages. Findings from both studies will inform whether broader use of these types of strategies can prevent abusive head trauma and save lives.

## Expanding The Reach And Accessibility Of Child Maltreatment Prevention Strategies

Strategies that effectively prevent child maltreatment and promote healthy child development are available but typically provided only to families with known risks. DVP supports the development and evaluation of approaches that increase the accessibility of evidence-based strategies and help all parents develop positive parenting behaviors. For instance, DVP is developing *Essentials for Parenting Toddlers and Preschoolers*, which uses a web-based platform with videos, interactive activities, and other resources to help parents of children aged 2–4 years develop safe, stable, and nurturing relationships with their children. DVP is also working with partners to evaluate the implementation in Pitt County, North Carolina and Berrien County, Michigan of *Triple P*, which is an evidence-based system of strategies for communities to enhance parents' abilities to raise their children in safe, loving, and engaging environments. The goal of the *Triple P* study is to identify and address barriers to widespread use of effective strategies. DVP also is examining strategies to prevent child maltreatment through other service delivery infrastructures. For example, *Early Head Start* (EHS) as a primary prevention strategy for child abuse and neglect is being examined by researchers at Portland State University to determine its impact on specific subgroups of children and families; how children in EHS and controls differ on timing, type, severity or chronicity of maltreatment experienced; and what characteristics of the program are associated with better outcomes. Researchers at Tulane University are evaluating the effects of two interventions (*Triple P-Level 2* and *Play Nicely*) versus usual care among parents receiving Women, Infants, and Children (WIC) services on parenting behaviors linked with child physical abuse. Finally, DVP supports formative research about how to better engage fathers in effective parenting and child maltreatment prevention programs, including an evaluation of *Fathers Supporting Success* in Preschoolers by researchers at Queens College and an evaluation of Engaging Fathers by researchers at Washington University. All of this research can help understand how to increase access to prevention approaches that work to prevent child maltreatment.

## Preventing Suicide With Connectedness

Suicide is a leading cause of death, but very little is known about how to effectively prevent it. DVP is leading efforts to better understand whether increasing social connectedness for at-risk individuals can lower the risk for suicide. DVP works with researchers at the University of Michigan to evaluate the *Links to Enhancing Teens' Connectedness* (*LET's CONNECT*) program, which focuses on youth aged 12–15 years who are at elevated risk for suicidal behavior due to low interpersonal connectedness, a recent history of bullying others, or a recent history of being bullied. *Let's Connect* teams adolescents with community and natural mentors to actively facilitate and support the adolescents' engagement with community organizations and activities to decrease the risk for suicide. Researchers at the University of Rochester are receiving funding to evaluate *The Senior Connection*, a suicide prevention strategy designed for older adults who are socially disconnected or feel that they are a burden on others. This strategy pairs these at-risk seniors with peer volunteers with the goal of increasing connectedness and decreasing suicide risk. This research is ground-breaking and could help reduce suicides among vulnerable groups.

## Evaluating Economic And Environmental Change Approaches To Prevent Violence

The social, economic, and physical characteristics of neighborhoods and communities influence the likelihood of violence, but little is known about the effectiveness of strategies to address these broader community risk factors. DVP's research is addressing this gap. For example, researchers at the University of Pittsburgh are receiving funding to evaluate the impact of a community economic development initiative on rates of youth violence and crime in urban neighborhoods. DVP is also supporting the RAND Corporation to evaluate the effects of school choice and school finance reform on community violence. DVP is working with researchers at ICF Macro to evaluate the impact of Colorado's state-supervised, county-administered Temporary Assistance to Needy Families program on child maltreatment and other child health outcomes over a 20 year period. Results of these research projects will inform strategies that strengthen the health and safety of communities.

## Comprehensive Youth Violence Prevention In High Risk Communities

Youth violence is caused by numerous factors, and its prevention requires multiple strategies that are systematically identified and implemented by many community partners. DVP's Academic Centers of Excellence in Youth Violence Prevention (ACEs) connect academic and community partners to implement and evaluate strategies to prevent violence in high-risk neighborhoods. The ACEs are taking the best available research evidence, implementing these strategies as part of a comprehensive approach, and then assessing their impact on assault, homicide, and other youth violence outcomes. The ACEs are a catalyst for prevention efforts in the communities that they serve. Their development and evaluation of innovative partnerships and prevention strategies are also creating new approaches that other communities can utilize and informing how national reductions in youth violence can be achieved.

## Family Approaches To Preventing Intimate Partner Violence

Family environments can create risks for or buffers against future violence. DVP is evaluating a number of innovative approaches to help at-risk individuals and families stop violence before it starts. DVP is providing funding to researchers at SUNY Stony Brook to conduct a randomized controlled trial of *Couple Care for Parents*, which is a self-directed program that builds healthy relationship skills of parents with newborns in order to reduce the potential of partner violence in the relationship. Researchers at the Boston VA Research Institute are receiving funding to evaluate *PTSD-Focused Relationship Enhancement Therapy*, which is a group-based approach for returning veterans from Iraq or Afghanistan and their partners and addresses PTSD symptoms, anger, and problem-solving skills. Researchers at John Jay College are being supported to examine the long-term impact of a preschool family intervention (which showed promise in reducing early childhood risk factors for delinquency and peer violence) on sexual and dating violence experiences in adolescence and young adulthood. University of North Carolina researchers are evaluating *Moms and Teens for Safe Dates*, which is a dating abuse primary prevention strategy for teens exposed to adult intimate partner violence in their homes. Findings from these studies will inform ways to act early to prevent the occurrence of dating and intimate partner violence and promote health.

## Preventing Sexual Violence Among Youth

Sexual violence is a pervasive problem that has broad and long-lasting impacts on health, yet we lack effective prevention strategies. DVP is supporting the University of Kentucky to conduct a population-based, state-wide randomized controlled trial of *Green Dot* in 26 high schools. *Green Dot* is a comprehensive bystander approach focused on the primary prevention of teen sexual and dating violence that uses social norms change strategies and skills training for peer leaders. Researchers at the University of Illinois at Urbana-Champaign are receiving support to conduct a randomized controlled trial of *Second Step: Student Success Through Prevention* in 34 middle schools. This classroom-based curriculum is implemented throughout 6th, 7th, and 8th grade and addresses the shared underlying risk and protective factors for bullying, sexual harassment, and dating aggression. In a second randomized controlled trail, University of Illinois at Urbana-Champaign researchers are comparing Second Step and a gender-enhanced *Second Step/Shifting Boundaries* program on violence perpetration, bystander behavior, and peer attitudes about violence. DVP also is working with Safe Place to evaluate *Expect Respect Support Groups* in preventing sexual and dating violence among at-risk middle and high school youth. Researchers at Rutgers University are receiving support to investigate the effectiveness of *SCREAM Theater*, a bystander intervention focused on reducing sexual violence among college students. This research will provide critical knowledge about strategies that stop sexual violence.

## Screening For Intimate Partner Violence

Many professional organizations recommend screening all women for intimate partner violence in primary care settings as a way to identify potential victims and to prevent the negative health outcomes of partner violence. Whether screening leads to better health, help-seeking, or prevents the recurrence of violence is less clear. Previous research by DVP examining whether screening for intimate partner violence and giving women information on partner violence resources improved health found no differences between participants who included women who were screened and provided a resource list, women who were not screened but given a resource list, and a control group. DVP is currently funding the Collaborative Research Unit at Stroger Hospital to evaluate the impact of screening for these participants within a 3-year period. Results can inform strategies to identify and support women experiencing intimate partner violence.

## Promoting Healthy Teen Relationships

Teen dating violence has significant negative effects on short-and long-term mental and physical health, and unhealthy teen relationships increase the risk for adult intimate partner violence. DVP developed *Dating Matters*—a comprehensive teen dating violence prevention program for youth, their parents, educators, and the neighborhoods in which they live. The program engages local health departments and reinforces skills taught to parents and youth through evidence-based programs with educator training and a communication campaign that uses social media and text messages. *Dating Matters* is being delivered in approximately 45 middle schools across 4 high-risk, urban communities and is being evaluated for its effectiveness in reducing the risk for physical, emotional, and sexual violence among teens and its cost effectiveness. This work will help guide and strengthen national efforts to stop dating violence.

# Help Others Be Violence-Free

The actions of one young person can greatly influence the actions of others. Youth can help prevent violence by speaking out and letting others know that violence is never okay. Implementation steps include:

- Help others be violence-free, and support those who have been hurt by violence. Young people are encouraged to not just wait and watch when violence is about to happen or is occurring around them. When youth see that their friends are getting upset, they can help them calm down and deal with the situation in a nonviolent way. Whenever it is safe to do so, youth can stop an argument from getting violent and let others know that they do not agree with bullying or other forms of violence. Young people should get help from others, like trusted adults, especially when it is not safe to address the problem on their own. It is also important for youth to support others who have been victims of violence so that they do not continue to be victimized or become violent themselves.

- Show others how to stay safe. By avoiding alcohol, drugs, or any form of violence, youth can increase their own safety and health and be positive models for their peers. Youth can also encourage their peers to make safe and healthy choices. When minors resolve conflicts in nonviolent ways and without involving weapons, they help keep themselves, their friends and families, their schools, and their neighborhoods safe.

- Get involved in violence prevention work. Young people can become involved in or initiate violence prevention work in their schools or communities. Having young people involved helps to ensure that violence prevention efforts are focusing on the right issues and working in ways that will engage youth. These are also opportunities for youth to build and share their experiences, skills, and talents to help others and to make connections with other nonviolent peers. Youth-led activities can help raise support for youth violence prevention among other youth and adults.

# Seizing The Opportunity And Responsibility To Prevent Youth Violence

The advances in our knowledge about youth violence and effective prevention strategies give us the opportunity to do more than simply wait and respond when violence occurs. We have learned how to proactively stop youth violence before our young people die or are injured. We have a responsibility to our young people and communities to use the evidence based prevention approaches that are already available and to continue research to expand our ability to stop youth violence before it starts. This work includes ensuring that prevention is a prominent element of a community's approach to violence and implemented prevention activities are based on what works. Communities are more likely to have an impact on youth violence and save money by using evidence-based prevention approaches over unproven ones. Existing knowledge about youth violence gives us the tools to act today and a solid foundation to continue to develop and test innovative prevention approaches that benefit all communities.

Part of the opportunity and responsibility to prevent youth violence includes activating, integrating, and utilizing public health professionals. They have the expertise and skills to strengthen communities' efforts to prevent youth violence. By partnering with and complementing the work of other sectors, including law enforcement, education, social services, and medical systems as well as faith-based, media, non-profit, and businesses, public health can contribute to and help lead the advancement of youth violence prevention activities. No matter who we are—community residents and leaders; public health practitioners; parents, teachers and others who work with youth; or young people—we all have an important role and actions we can take to protect America's youth and to help prevent youth violence.

# Chapter 41
# When Parents Fight

## When Parents Disagree

All couples argue from time to time. They might disagree about important things like finances, careers, or major family decisions. Or they might disagree about little things that don't seem that important—like what's for dinner or what time someone gets home.

Sometimes parents stay calm when they disagree. They allow each other a chance to listen and to talk. But many times when parents disagree, things can get heated.

It can be easy to jump to conclusions when you hear parents arguing. Thoughts might pop into your head like, "Does this mean they don't love each other anymore?" Or, "Are they going to get a divorce?" But arguments don't always mean the worst. Most of the time, they're just a way to let off steam when parents have a bad day, don't feel well, or are under a lot of stress. Like you, when parents get upset they might yell, cry, or say things they don't really mean.

## It's OK For Parents To Argue Sometimes

It's natural for people to have different feelings, opinions, or approaches to things. Talking about these differences is a first step in working toward a solution. People in a family need to be able to tell each other how they feel and what they think, even when they disagree.

Most people who live together in a family argue about small things—like if the way you do something is different from how a brother, sister, or parent does it. Watching how parents resolve differences can give you some important information about how you handle conflict, and how you might handle arguments in the future.

About This Chapter: Text in this chapter is excerpted from "When Parents Argue," © 1995–2016. The Nemours Foundation/KidsHealth®. Reprinted with permission.

Most of the time, arguments are over quickly, parents apologize and make up, and the family settles back into its usual routine.

## When Fighting Goes Too Far

Sometimes when parents fight, there's too much yelling and screaming, name calling, and too many harsh things said. Although some parents may do this, it's not OK to treat people in the family with disrespect, use degrading or insulting language, or yell and scream at them.

Occasionally fighting goes too far and includes pushing and shoving, throwing things, or hitting. Even if no one is physically hurt, an argument has gone too far when one parent uses threats to try to control the other through fear. It's never OK if a parent does things like these:

- threatens to hurt someone

- destroys the other's property

- threatens to commit suicide

- threatens to leave the other parent

- threatens to report the other parent to protective services

When fights get physical or involve threats, it's usually a sign that the people fighting could do with some help controlling themselves and managing their anger. This may mean speaking to a doctor, therapist, or religious leader or calling a helpline.

## What About You?

It's hard to hear parents yelling at each other. Seeing them upset and out of control can throw you off—aren't adults, especially parents, supposed to be the calm, composed, mature ones in a family? How much parents' fighting bothers you might depend on how often it happens, how loud or intense things get, or whether parents argue in front of other people.

It's natural to worry about a parent who may feel hurt by what the other parent says. Maybe you worry that one parent could become angry enough to lose control and physically hurt the other. With all this extra mental and emotional turmoil, you may start to feel the signs of stress, like being tearful, getting stomachaches or headaches, or having trouble sleeping. If parents' arguments start to get in the way of how well you eat, sleep, or pay attention in school, talk to a school counselor or teacher.

It can be especially upsetting if parents are arguing about you. But your parents' arguments are never your fault. Parents are responsible for their own actions and behaviors, no matter how much they are provoked by another person.

## What You Can Do

If you feel that your parents' fighting is getting too much for you and you're stressed out about it, it's time to take action. You could try talking to one or both of your parents about their arguing. They may not even realize how upset you are until you tell them how their arguments affect you. If this doesn't work, you could try talking to another family member to help you figure out what to do—or go to your school counselor or doctor.

If the fighting goes too far in your family (or that of someone you know), let an adult know what's going on. Talking to relatives, a school counselor, a favorite teacher, or any adult you trust can be helpful. Sometimes parents who fight can get so out of control that they hurt each other or other family members. If this happens, letting someone else know will allow the family to get help and kids to be protected from harmful fighting.

Family members can get help from counselors and therapists. This can help them learn to listen to each other and talk about feelings and differences without arguments getting heated. Though it may take some work, time, and practice, people in families can learn to get along better.

## Happy, Healthy Families

If your family argues from time to time, try not to worry: No family is perfect. Even in the happiest home, problems come up and people argue. Usually the family members involved get what's bothering them out in the open and talk about it. Hopefully, they reach some compromise or agreement. Everyone feels better and life can get back to normal.

Being part of a family means everyone pitches in and tries to make life better for each other. Arguments happen and that's OK—it's all part of learning how to live with each other and get along. Figuring out how to resolve conflicts by talking things out or learning when other people need their space can help you later in your life, too.

# Chapter 42

# Afterschool Programs

Afterschool programs (sometimes called OST or Out-of-School Time) serve children and youth of all ages, and encompass a broad range of focus areas including academic support, mentoring, youth development, arts, and sports and recreation. The activities in which children and youth engage while outside of school hours are critical to their development, highlighting the need for quality afterschool programs in all communities. The demand for afterschool programs is strong; current estimates suggest that nearly 10 million children and youth participate in afterschool programs annually, 10 million in summer camps, and 6 million in 4-H programs alone.

High quality afterschool programs generate positive outcomes for youth including improved academic performance, classroom behavior, and health and nutrition. Communities and businesses also benefit when youth have safe and productive ways to spend their time while their parents are at work. Several Federal agencies provide support and resources to afterschool programs to help promote positive outcomes for youth.

## Benefits For Youth, Families, And Communities

Effective afterschool programs bring a wide range of benefits to youth, families and communities. Afterschool programs can boost academic performance, reduce risky behaviors, promote physical health, and provide a safe, structured environment for the children of working parents.

- Attending afterschool programs can improve students' academic performance. A national evaluation found that over 40 percent of students attending 21st Century Community

About This Chapter: This chapter includes text excerpted from "Afterschool Program," Youth.gov, September 30, 2011. Reviewed November 2016.

Learning Center programs improved their reading and math grades, and that those who attended more regularly were more likely to make gains.

- Effective afterschool programs can improve classroom behavior, school attendance, academic aspirations, and can reduce the likelihood that a student will drop out.

- Participation in afterschool programs has been associated with reduced drug use and criminal behavior.

- Afterschool programs can play an important role in encouraging physical activity and good dietary habits. Participation in afterschool programs has been associated with positive health outcomes, including reduced obesity.

- Working families and businesses also derive benefits from afterschool programs that ensure that youth have a safe place to go while parents are at work. Parents concerned about their children's afterschool care miss an average of eight days of work per year, and this decreased worker productivity costs businesses up to $300 billion annually.

# Activities

Afterschool activities can vary widely depending on factors including age, background, and the community of participating youth. Research on afterschool programming finds that the most effective activities adapt to individual and small group needs. Furthermore, programming should be as engaging as possible, incorporating hands-on activities and connecting with students' interests and experiences.

Different types of afterschool activities include:

**Academics and Enrichment**

These types of activities are intended to build on and enhance student learning outside of class time. They can take the form of more traditional instruction, complete with assessments, or more interactive activities intended to actively engage youth. These activities should be well aligned with what students are learning during the school day.

**Community Service Projects**

Community service projects provide an enriching experience for youth that connect them to their community and instill feelings of empowerment. Furthermore, these activities can provide valuable work experience, particularly for youth from disadvantaged backgrounds. The Corporation for National and Community Service provides resources to help plan community service projects for afterschool programs, including the Resource Center for Volunteer and Service Programs and the National Service-Learning Clearinghouse.

**Field Trips**

Field Trips are an exciting way to enrich a child's life outside of the normal classroom environment. They can include trips to museums, parks, zoos, aquariums, or any other local attraction that youth might find engaging and interesting.

**Physical Activity and Nutrition**

Afterschool programs are in a unique position to improve youth health outcomes, as they often serve populations most at risk for adverse health outcomes and occur at a time of day when many youth are traditionally inactive. Such activities can help youth make better nutritional decisions and promote physical activity while increasing self-confidence and emotional well-being.

# Health And Nutrition

Afterschool programs are well-positioned to promote health and nutrition among young people because these programs:

- Serve many groups of children most at risk for being overweight, specifically minorities and those in poverty

- Occur during a time of day when children are likely to be sedentary if not given active options

- Reach children at the developmental stage when they are forming the health patterns they will carry into adulthood

- Provide meals and snacks that can serve as nutritious examples for dietary habits

- Act as liaisons to parents who make critical nutrition and physical activity decisions for their children

- Have experience in making learning fun and modifying lessons for the needs of their students and clients

- Offer a supportive, safe environment in which children can feel comfortable trying new activities and building new skills; and

- Are led by caring adults who can act as role models with positive influence on children's health and nutrition choices

Afterschool programs can encourage healthy outcomes for youth by providing opportunities for physical activity, promoting good nutrition, and engaging parents to encourage healthy choices at home.

# Chapter 43
# Conflict Resolution

Conflict is a normal, natural part of human relationships. People will not agree about everything all the time. In and of itself, conflict is not necessarily a negative thing. When handled constructively it can help people to stand up for themselves and others, and work together to achieve a mutually satisfactory solution. But if conflict is handled poorly it can cause anger, hurt, divisiveness and more serious problems. This chapter discusses how to deal with conflict in a constructive manner.

## Sources Of Conflict

There can be many causes or reasons for conflict. However, some of the most common include:

- **Personal differences** such as values, ethics, personalities, age, education, gender, social and economic status, cultural background, temperament, health, religion, political beliefs, etc.

- **A clash of ideas, choices, or actions.** For instance, conflict can occur when people have incompatible goals, when they are in direct competition, or even when they have different work styles.

- Finally, **poor communication** or miscommunication is one of the biggest causes of conflict.

About This Chapter: This chapter includes text excerpted from "Conflict Resolution," National Oceanic and Atmospheric Administration (NOAA), October 14, 2012. Reviewed November 2016.

# Preventing Conflict

While it isn't possible to prevent all conflict, there are steps that you can take to try to keep conflict to a minimum. One way to manage conflict is to prevent it from occurring in the first place. Preventing conflict is not the same as avoiding conflict. Preventing conflict means behaving and communicating in a way that averts needless conflicts.

Consider the following tips:

- **Respect differences.** Many conflicts arise from differences in gender, generations, cultures, values, etc. We live in an increasingly diverse world. Learn to respect and celebrate peoples' differences and their opinions.

- **Treat others as you'd like to be treated.** Regardless of your personal opinion of someone, be professional, courteous, respectful, and tolerant, even when you're frustrated. If a person treats you disrespectfully, calmly tell them you do not appreciate it. Do not exacerbate the situation by retaliating with inappropriate behavior or comments.

- **Keep negative opinions to yourself**—Most people are put off by hearing negative comments about others—especially if it's about personal issue. In the workplace, this may lead to disciplinary action. Friends and acquaintances may be equally "turned off" by negative comments about someone, particularly if they feel they are being drawn into a conflict or being asked to take sides. If you need to vent about a personal issue, do so outside of the workplace, keep it to a close, trusted friend or a loved one and keep it to a minimum.

- **Keep your distance**—Unfortunately, this is often easier said than done. Often the conflicts arise with those who are closest to us. It is often easier to get along if you respect one another's privacy and boundaries. Taking a break from each other can go along way in keeping the peace.

# Resolving Conflict

Sometimes, conflict cannot—or should not—be avoided. Knowing how to deal with conflict is important for anyone. However, often people have not been given the tools to effectively deal with conflict. Consider the following tips:

- **Address the issue early.** The longer you let an issue fester, the more time you waste and the greater chance you have of it spiraling into other problems.

- **Address the issue privately.** Set up a time to talk in a private place, where you won't be overheard or interrupted. Speak to the person with whom you have the conflict and try to resolve the issue one-on-one before involving others.

- **Expect discomfort.** You may have to say up front: "Although this is uncomfortable for me, if I don't address this, I'm afraid we will not meet our goal."

- **Be specific and objective.** Identify the specific issue at hand and the effect it is having. Avoid generalizing statements such as "always," "ever" or "never." Stick to the subject; try not to digress into broad personality issues or revive past issues.

- **Focus on the outcome.** Don't dwell on problems or blame. Keep the spotlight on finding solutions and how you will reach the desired outcomes. "In order to reach the goal of X, I think we need to do Y."

- **Be open.** Doing so establishes an atmosphere of mutual respect and cooperation. Listen to and consider others' opinions, points of view and ideas. Understand and appreciate that they think differently than you and may bring a greater, or different, understanding to the table that will help resolve the problem more quickly and effectively.

- **Respond constructively.** Let the other person know you value what he or she is saying, even if you don't agree. Try to avoid responding negatively or directively, for example criticizing, ridiculing, dismissing, diverting (talking about yourself rather than about what the other person has said) or rejecting the other person or what they are saying.

- **Know your triggers.** Learn to recognize your personal warning signs for anger and figure out the ways that work for best for you to constructively control your anger.

- **Maintain a sense of humor.** Be willing to laugh, including at yourself. Maintaining a sense of humor can relieve stress and tension, and help get you and others through a difficult time.

- **Learn to compromise.** Compromise is important in any relationship. If you disagree on an issue, discuss the problem calmly, allow each person to explain his or her point of view, and look for ways to meet each other in the middle.

- **Don't attempt to resolve conflict when tempers are flaring.** During an argument, often no one can agree on a reasonable solution. If that is the case, agree to take a break and come back to the problem later, when you have had time to settle down and think about the issue.

- **Know when to retreat.** The conflict resolution process will not always work. The level of the skills of some people may not be at the point where they can be full partners in this process. For example, you may have a spouse who does not want to, or know how to, solve the problem. You may also have a conflict with a coworker, boss or higher-up who is known for irrational outbursts. You must take all these factors into consideration and know when it may be more appropriate for you to cut your losses and retreat.

- **Practice forgiveness.** There may be times when someone makes a mistake or says or does something hurtful—whether intentionally or unintentionally. While it's okay to be angry, it's also important to let go of the anger and move on. On a personal level, it is healthier to let go of negative emotions like stress and anger. And it's difficult to maintain a good relationship if you can't get past these feelings.

# Mutual Conflict Resolution

In most cases you should be able to resolve conflicts by working with others involved. Here are some steps to consider:

- **Step One:** Identify the purpose and importance of the conflict—and your mutual desire to solve it.

- **Step Two:** Takes turns listening to each other's side. This is a very important step and one that requires good listening skills.

- **Step Three:** Once all the issues are discussed, repeat and summarize what was said.

- **Step Four:** Ask questions as needed and encourage others to do the same. Do you understand their point of view? Are you sure they understand yours? Clarify as needed.

- **Step Five:** No matter how intense the conflict, you should always find issues or points that you agree upon.

- **Step Six:** Next, list ALL solutions—even those that may seem unrealistic, unreasonable, or wrong.

- **Step Seven:** Review all the possible solutions and highlight those you find mutually acceptable. Hopefully you will have at least one or two that you agree upon.

- **Step Eight:** Choose the one (or few) that you agree will work best.

- **Step Nine:** Put a plan into action. What steps will you take to implement? How will you review progress?

By creating step-by-step guidelines and mutually agreed upon solutions and action plans, you should be able to minimize conflict and achieve desired goals.

# Dealing Constructively With Anger

Conflict can result in anger. Anger is a normal human emotion ranging from annoyance to absolute rage. Each person's anger "triggers" are different, some may get angry at a friend's behavior, other causes of anger can be more serious—such as personal problems or a previous traumatic experience. In and of itself, anger is not necessarily a problem—when focused appropriately it can help people to stand up for themselves and others. But if anger is channeled in negative, inappropriate ways it can cause problems. Consider the following ideas to help deal constructively with anger:

- Anger is a strong emotion, and isn't always easy to control. Two crucial skills in managing anger are self-awareness and self-control. Try to recognize and identify your feelings, especially anger. Once the feeling is identified you can then think about the appropriate response.

- **Self-awareness** is being conscious of thoughts and feelings. Examine how and why you are feeling angry to better understand and manage these feelings. For example, ask yourself questions such as "why am I angry?" or "what is making me feel this way?" to assist in self-analysis. Learn to recognize your personal warning signs for anger.

- **Self-control** means stopping and considering actions before taking them. Learn to stop and think before you act or speak in anger. For example, envision a stop sign when you are angry—and to take the time to think about how to react. Explore techniques to calm down such as counting backwards from ten to one, deep breathing, or just walking away.

- **Relax.** Try relaxation exercises, such as breathing deeply from the diaphragm (the belly, not the chest) and slowly repeating a calming word or phrase like "take it easy." Or to think of relaxing experiences, such as sitting on a beach or walking through a forest.

- **Think positively.** Remind yourself that no one is out to get you, you are just experiencing some of the rough spots of daily life.

- **Problem-solve.** Identify the specific problem that is causing the anger and approach it head-on—even if the problem does not have a quick solution.

- **Communicate with others.** Angry people tend to jump to conclusions and speak without thinking about the consequences of what they are saying. Slow down and think carefully about what you want to say. Listen carefully to what the other person is saying.

- **Manage stress.** Set aside personal time to deal with the daily stresses of work, activities, and family. Ideas include: listening to music, writing in a journal, exercising, meditating, or talking about your feelings with someone you trust.

- **Change the scene.** A change of environment may help reduce angry feelings. For example, if your co-workers or friends are angry frequently and/or make you angry, consider spending time with people who may contribute more to your self-confidence and well-being.

- **Find a distraction.** If you can't seem to let your anger go, it can help to do something distracting, for example, read or watch television or a movie.

- **Set a good example.** If you are teaching your child to control their anger, make sure you practice what you preach. Show by example how you manage your own anger.

# Chapter 44
# Is Your Relationship A Healthy One?

Sometimes it feels impossible to find someone who's right for you—and who thinks *you're* right for him or her! So when it happens, you're usually so psyched that you don't even mind when your little brother finishes all the ice cream or your English teacher chooses the one day when you didn't do your reading to give you a pop quiz.

It's totally normal to look at the world through rose-colored glasses in the early stages of a relationship. But for some people, those rose-colored glasses turn into blinders that keep them from seeing that a relationship isn't as healthy as it should be.

## What Makes A Healthy Relationship?

Hopefully, you and your significant other are treating each other well. Not sure if that's the case? Take a step back from the dizzying sensation of being swept off your feet and think about whether your relationship has these seven qualities:

- **Mutual respect.** Does he or she get how cool you are and why? (Watch out if the answer to the first part is yes but only because you're acting like someone you're not!) The key is that your BF or GF is into you for who you are—for your great sense of humor, your love of reality TV, etc. Does your partner listen when you say you're not comfortable doing something and then back off right away? Respect in a relationship means that each person values who the other is and understands—and would never challenge—the other person's boundaries.

---

- **Trust.** You're talking with a guy from French class and your boyfriend walks by. Does he completely lose his cool or keep walking because he knows you'd never cheat on him? It's OK to get a little jealous sometimes—jealousy is a natural emotion. But how a person reacts when feeling jealous is what matters. There's no way you can have a healthy relationship if you don't trust each other.

- **Honesty.** This one goes hand-in-hand with trust because it's tough to trust someone when one of you isn't being honest. Have you ever caught your girlfriend in a major lie? Like she told you that she had to work on Friday night but it turned out she was at the movies with her friends? The next time she says she has to work, you'll have a lot more trouble believing her and the trust will be on shaky ground.

- **Support.** It's not just in bad times that your partner should support you. Some people are great when your whole world is falling apart but can't take being there when things are going right (and vice versa). In a healthy relationship, your significant other is there with a shoulder to cry on when you find out your parents are getting divorced **and** to celebrate with you when you get the lead in a play.

- **Fairness/equality.** You need to have give-and-take in your relationship, too. Do you take turns choosing which new movie to see? As a couple, do you hang out with your partner's friends as often as you hang out with yours? It's not like you have to keep a running count and make sure things are exactly even, of course. But you'll know if it isn't a pretty fair balance. Things get bad really fast when a relationship turns into a power struggle, with one person fighting to get his or her way all the time.

- **Separate identities.** In a healthy relationship, everyone needs to make compromises. But that doesn't mean you should feel like you're losing out on being yourself. When you started going out, you both had your own lives (families, friends, interests, hobbies, etc.) and that shouldn't change. Neither of you should have to pretend to like something you don't, or give up seeing your friends, or drop out of activities you love. And you also should feel free to keep developing new talents or interests, making new friends, and moving forward.

- **Good communication.** You've probably heard lots of stuff about how men and women don't seem to speak the same language. We all know how many different meanings the little phrase "no, nothing's wrong" can have, depending on who's saying it! But what's important is to ask if you're not sure what he or she means, and speak honestly and openly so that the miscommunication is avoided in the first place. Never keep a feeling bottled up because you're afraid it's not what your BF or GF wants to hear or because you worry about sounding silly. And if you need some time to think something through before you're ready to talk about it, the right person will give you some space to do that if you ask for it.

## What's An Unhealthy Relationship?

A relationship is unhealthy when it involves mean, disrespectful, controlling, or abusive behavior. Some people live in homes with parents who fight a lot or abuse each other—emotionally, verbally, or physically. For some people who have grown up around this kind of behavior it can almost seem normal or OK. **It's not!** Many of us learn from watching and imitating the people close to us. So someone who has lived around violent or disrespectful behavior may not have learned how to treat others with kindness and respect or how to expect the same treatment.

Qualities like kindness and respect are absolute requirements for a healthy relationship. Someone who doesn't yet have this part down may need to work on it with a trained therapist before he or she is ready for a relationship. Meanwhile, even though you might feel bad or feel for someone who's been mistreated, you need to take care of yourself—it's not healthy to stay in a relationship that involves abusive behavior of any kind.

## Warning Signs

When a boyfriend or girlfriend uses verbal insults, mean language, nasty putdowns, gets physical by hitting or slapping, or forces someone into sexual activity, it's a sign of verbal, emotional, or physical abuse.

Ask yourself, does my boyfriend or girlfriend:

- get angry when I don't drop everything for him or her?
- criticize the way I look or dress, and say I'll never be able to find anyone else who would date me?
- keep me from seeing friends or from talking to any other guys or girls?
- want me to quit an activity, even though I love it?
- ever raise a hand when angry, like he or she is about to hit me?
- try to force me to go further sexually than I want to?

These aren't the only questions you can ask yourself. If you can think of any way in which your boyfriend or girlfriend is trying to control you, make you feel bad about yourself, isolate you from the rest of your world, or—this is a big one—harm you physically or sexually, then it's time to get out, *fast*. Let a trusted friend or family member know what's going on and make sure you're safe.

It can be tempting to make excuses or misinterpret violence, possessiveness, or anger as an expression of love. But even if you know that the person hurting you loves you, it is not healthy. No one deserves to be hit, shoved, or forced into anything he or she doesn't want to do.

## Why Are Some Relationships So Difficult?

Ever heard about how it's hard for someone to love you when you don't love yourself? It's a big relationship roadblock when one or both people struggle with self-esteem problems. Your girlfriend or boyfriend isn't there to make you feel good about yourself if you can't do that on your own. Focus on being happy with yourself, and don't take on the responsibility of worrying about someone else's happiness.

What if you feel that your girlfriend or boyfriend needs too much from you? If the relationship feels like a burden or a drag instead of a joy, it might be time to think about whether it's a healthy match for you. Someone who's not happy or secure may have trouble being a healthy relationship partner.

Also, intense relationships can be hard for some teenagers. Some are so focused on their own developing feelings and responsibilities that they don't have the emotional energy it takes to respond to someone else's feelings and needs in a close relationship. Don't worry if you're just not ready yet. You will be, and you can take all the time you need.

Ever notice that some teen relationships don't last very long? It's no wonder—you're still growing and changing every day, and it can be tough to put two people together whose identities are both still in the process of forming. You two might seem perfect for each other at first, but that can change. If you try to hold on to the relationship anyway, there's a good chance it will turn sour. Better to part as friends than to stay in something that you've outgrown or that no longer feels right for one or both of you. And before you go looking for amour from that hottie from French class, respect your current beau by breaking things off before you make your move.

Relationships can be one of the best—and most challenging—parts of your world. They can be full of fun, romance, excitement, intense feelings, and occasional heartache, too. Whether you're single or in a relationship, remember that it's good to be choosy about who you get close to. If you're still waiting, take your time and get to know plenty of people.

Think about the qualities you value in a friendship and see how they match up with the ingredients of a healthy relationship. Work on developing those good qualities in yourself—they make you a lot more attractive to others. And if you're already part of a pair, make sure the relationship you're in brings out the best in both of you.

# Chapter 45

# How To Help A Friend Who Is Abused At Home

Here are some ways to help a friend who is being abused:

- **Set up a time to talk**. Try to make sure you have privacy and won't be distracted or interrupted.

- **Let your friend know you're concerned about her safety.** Be honest. Tell her about times when you were worried about her. Help her see that what she's going through is not right. Let her know you want to help.

- **Be supportive.** Listen to your friend. Keep in mind that it may be very hard for her to talk about the abuse. Tell her that she is not alone, and that people want to help.

- **Offer specific help.** You might say you are willing to just listen, to help her with childcare, or to provide transportation, for example.

- **Don't place shame, blame, or guilt on your friend.** Don't say, "You just need to leave." Instead, say something like, "I get scared thinking about what might happen to you." Tell her you understand that her situation is very difficult.

- **Help her make a safety plan.** Safety planning includes picking a place to go and packing important items.

- **Encourage your friend to talk to someone who can help.** Offer to help her find a local domestic violence agency. Offer to go with her to the agency, the police, or court.

About This Chapter: Text in this chapter begins with excerpts from "Get Help For Violence," Office on Women's Health (OWH), U.S. Department of Health and Human Services (HHS), September 4, 2015; Text under the heading "Help Someone In An Unhealthy Relationship: Quick Tips" is excerpted from "Help Someone In An Unhealthy Relationship: Quick Tips," Office of Disease Prevention and Health Promotion (ODPHP), U.S. Department of Health and Human Services (HHS), March 22, 2016.

- **If your friend decides to stay, continue to be supportive.** Your friend may decide to stay in the relationship, or she may leave and then go back many times. It may be hard for you to understand, but people stay in abusive relationships for many reasons. Be supportive, no matter what your friend decides to do.

- **Encourage your friend to do things outside of the relationship.** It's important for her to see friends and family.

- **If your friend decides to leave, continue to offer support.** Even though the relationship was abusive, she may feel sad and lonely once it is over. She also may need help getting services from agencies or community groups.

- **Keep in mind that you can't "rescue" your friend.** She has to be the one to decide it's time to get help. Support her no matter what her decision.

- **Let your friend know that you will always be there no matter what.**

# Help Someone In An Unhealthy Relationship: Quick Tips

It can be hard to know what to do when someone you care about is in a controlling or violent relationship. These tips can help.

## Watch for signs of abuse.

Relationship violence can take many forms. Make a list of anything you notice that doesn't seem right. For example, watch for signs of:

- Controlling behavior, like demanding all of your loved one's time

- Physical abuse, like bruises or cuts

- Emotional abuse, like put-downs or name-calling

## Find out about local resources.

Before you talk with your friend or family member, call 1-800-799-SAFE (1-800-799-7233) to get the address and phone number of the nearest domestic violence agency. This way, you'll be able to share the information if the person is ready for it.

You can offer to help your friend or family member call the agency. You can also suggest visiting the domestic violence agency, talking to the police, or going to the doctor together.

## Set up a time to talk.

Make sure you can have your conversation in a safe, private place.

Keep in mind that your loved one's partner may have access to her cell phone or computer, so be careful about sharing information over text or email.

## Be specific about why you are worried.

Does your friend or loved one:

- Spend less time with friends or doing things he used to enjoy?
- Make excuses for his partner's behavior?
- Have unexplained cuts or bruises?

Does your friend or loved one's partner:

- Yell at or make fun of her?
- Try to control her by making all of the decisions?
- Check up on her when she's at work or school?
- Force her to do sexual things she doesn't want to do?
- Threaten to hurt himself if she ever breaks up with him?

Try to help your loved one understand that being treated this way isn't right. The more specific you can be, the better.

## Plan for safety.

People whose partners are controlling or violent may be in danger when they leave the relationship.

If your friend or loved one is ready to leave an abusive partner, help him make a plan for getting out of the relationship as safely as possible. A domestic violence counselor can help with making a safety plan.

If someone is in immediate danger, don't wait—call 911.

## Be patient.

Do your best to share your concerns with your friend or loved one—but understand that she will decide what's right for her, even if it doesn't make sense to you.

243

It can take time for someone to be ready to talk. Let her know that you are available to talk again whenever she is ready.

## Get help for yourself.

Watching someone you care about stay in an unhealthy relationship is hard. You can get support, too. Call 1-800-799-SAFE (1-800-799-7233).

# Chapter 46

# What Happens When Possible Abuse Or Neglect Is Reported

Any concerned person can report suspicions of child abuse or neglect. Most reports are made by "mandatory reporters"—people who are required by State law to report suspicions of child abuse and neglect. As of August 2012, statutes in approximately 18 States and Puerto Rico require any person who suspects child abuse or neglect to report it. These reports are generally received by child protective services (CPS) workers and are either "screened in" or "screened out." A report is screened in when there is sufficient information to suggest an investigation is warranted. A report may be screened out if there is not enough information on which to follow up or if the situation reported does not meet the State's legal definition of abuse or neglect. In these instances, the worker may refer the person reporting the incident to other community services or law enforcement for additional help.

## What Happens After A Report Is "Screened In"

CPS caseworkers, often called investigators or assessment workers, respond within a particular time period, which may be anywhere from a few hours to a few days, depending on the type of maltreatment alleged, the potential severity of the situation, and requirements under State law. They may speak with the parents and other people in contact with the child, such as doctors, teachers, or child care providers. They also may speak with the child, alone or in the presence of caregivers, depending on the child's age and level of risk. Children who are believed to be in immediate danger may be moved to a shelter, a foster home, or a relative's home during the investigation and while court proceedings are pending. An investigator also

About This Chapter: This chapter includes text excerpted from "How The Child Welfare System Works," Child Welfare Information Gateway, U.S. Department of Health and Human Services (HHS), February 2013. Reviewed November 2016.

engages the family, assessing strengths and needs and initiating connections to community resources and services.

Some jurisdictions now employ an alternative, or differential, response system. In these jurisdictions, when the risk to the children involved is considered low, the CPS caseworker focuses on assessing family strengths, resources, and difficulties and on identifying supports and services needed, rather than on gathering evidence to confirm the occurrence of abuse or neglect.

At the end of an investigation, CPS caseworkers typically make one of two findings—unsubstantiated (unfounded) or substantiated (founded). These terms vary from State to State. Typically, a finding of unsubstantiated means there is insufficient evidence for the worker to conclude that a child was abused or neglected, or what happened does not meet the legal definition of child abuse or neglect. A finding of substantiated typically means that an incident of child abuse or neglect, as defined by State law, is believed to have occurred. Some States have additional categories, such as "unable to determine," that suggest there was not enough evidence to either confirm or refute that abuse or neglect occurred.

The agency will initiate a court action if it determines that the authority of the juvenile court (through a child protection or dependency proceeding) is necessary to keep the child safe. To protect the child, the court can issue temporary orders placing the child in shelter care during the investigation, ordering services, or ordering certain individuals to have no contact with the child. At an adjudicatory hearing, the court hears evidence and decides whether maltreatment occurred and whether the child should be under the continuing jurisdiction of the court. The court then enters a disposition, either at that hearing or at a separate hearing, which may result in the court ordering a parent to comply with services necessary to alleviate the abuse or neglect. Orders can also contain provisions regarding visitation between the parent and the child, agency obligations to provide the parent with services, and services needed by the child.

# What Happens In Substantiated (Founded) Cases

If a child has been abused or neglected, the course of action depends on State policy, the severity of the maltreatment, an assessment of the child's immediate safety, the risk of continued or future maltreatment, the services available to address the family's needs, and whether the child was removed from the home and a court action to protect the child was initiated. The following general options are available:

- **No or low risk**—The family's case may be closed with no services if the maltreatment was a one-time incident, the child is considered to be safe, there is no or low risk of future incidents, and any services the family needs will not be provided through the child welfare agency but through other community based resources and service systems.

- **Low to moderate risk**—Referrals may be made to community-based or voluntary in-home child welfare services if the CPS worker believes the family would benefit from these services and the child's present and future safety would be enhanced. This may happen even when no abuse or neglect is found, if the family needs and is willing to participate in services.

- **Moderate to high risk**—The family may again be offered voluntary in-home services to address safety concerns and help reduce the risks. If these are refused, the agency may seek intervention by the juvenile dependency court. Once there is a judicial determination that abuse or neglect occurred, juvenile dependency court may require the family to cooperate with in-home services if it is believed that the child can remain safely at home while the family addresses the issues contributing to the risk of future maltreatment. If the child has been seriously harmed, is considered to be at high risk of serious harm, or the child's safety is threatened, the court may order the child's removal from the home or affirm the agency's prior removal of the child. The child may be placed with a relative or in foster care.

# Chapter 47
# Creating A Safety Plan

First, if you think that you are in an unhealthy relationship, you should talk to a parent/guardian, friend, counselor, doctor, teacher, coach or other trusted person about your relationship. Tell them why you think the relationship is unhealthy and exactly what the other person has done (hit, pressured you to have sex, tried to control you). If need be, this trusted adult can help you contact your parent/guardian, counselors, school security, or even the police about the violence. With help, you can get out of an unhealthy relationship.

Sometimes, leaving an abusive relationship can be dangerous, so it is very important for you to make a safety plan. Leaving the relationship will be a lot easier and safer if you have a plan.

Here are some tips on making your safety plan:

- Go to your doctor or hospital for treatment if you have been injured.

- Tell a trusted adult like a parent/guardian, counselor, doctor, teacher, or spiritual or community leader.

- Tell the person who is abusing you over the phone that you do not want to see him or her so they cannot touch you. Do this when a parent or guardian is home so you know you will be safe in your house.

- Use a diary to keep track of the date the violence happened, where you were, exactly what the person you are dating did, and exactly what effects it caused (such as bruises). This will be important if you need the police to order the person to stay away from you.

About This Chapter: Text in this chapter begins with excerpts from "In Relationships," Office on Women's Health (OWH), U.S. Department of Health and Human Services (HHS), September 22, 2009. Reviewed November 2016; Text beginning with the heading "If You Are A Victim Of Sexual Assault" is excerpted from "Help And Support For Victims," National Sex Offender Public Website (NSOPW), U.S. Department of Justice (DOJ), December 21, 2011. Reviewed November 2016.

- Avoid contact with the person.

- Spend time with your other friends, and avoid walking by yourself.

- Think of safe places to go in case of an emergency, like a police station or a public place like a restaurant or mall.

- Carry a cell phone, phone card, or money for a call in case you need to call for help. Use code words on the phone that you and your family decide on ahead of time. If you are in trouble, say the code word on the phone so that your family member knows you can't talk openly and need help right away.

- Call 911 right away if you are ever afraid that the person is following you or is going to hurt you.

- Keep domestic violence hotline numbers with you in a safe place or program them into your cell phone. The 24-hour National Domestic Violence Hotline is 1-800-799-SAFE (1-800-799-7233) or 1-800-787-3224 (TDD).

## If You Are A Victim Of Sexual Assault

- Try to get to a place where you feel safe.

- Reach out for support.

- Call someone you trust, such as a friend or a family member. You are not alone; there are people who can give you the support you need.

- Call the National Sexual Assault Hotline at 800-656-HOPE (800-656-4673)—your call is free and is anonymous and confidential.

- Seek medical attention as soon as possible. Medical care is important to address any injuries you may have and to protect against sexually transmitted diseases and pregnancy.

- Most important, know that the assault is not your fault.

## Seek Help Or Support

The national contacts below are available for anyone seeking information and resources about sexual abuse. In an emergency, please dial 9-1-1 for local assistance immediately.

- **Child Help National Child Abuse Hotline**

  By phone: 800-4-A-CHILD (800-422-4453)

- **Darkness to Light**

  By phone: 866-367-5444. Toll-free helpline for individuals living in the United States who need local information and resources about sexual abuse.

- **National Center for Missing and Exploited Children**

  By phone: 800-843-5678. Available 24 hours a day. This toll-free line is for reporting any information about missing or sexually exploited children to the police. This number is available throughout the United States, Mexico, and Canada. The TDD Hotline is 800-826-7653.

- **National Center for Victims of Crime**

  By phone: 800-394-2255. Toll-free helpline offers supportive counseling, practical information about crime and victimization, and referrals to local community resources, as well as skilled advocacy in the criminal justice and social service systems.

- **Rape, Abuse and Incest National Network**

  By phone: 800-656-4673. Toll-free National Sexual Assault Hotline.

# Chapter 48

# Self-Defense

Many people think of self-defense as a karate kick to the groin or jab in the eyes of an attacker. But self-defense actually means doing everything possible to avoid fighting someone who threatens or attacks you. Self-defense is all about using your smarts—not your fists.

## Use Your Head

People (guys as well as girls) who are threatened and fight back "in self-defense" actually risk making a situation worse. The attacker, who is already edgy and pumped up on adrenaline—and who knows what else—may become even more angry and violent. The best way to handle any attack or threat of attack is to try to get away. This way, you're least likely to be injured.

One way to avoid a potential attack before it happens is to trust your instincts. Your intuition, combined with your common sense, can help get you out of trouble. For example, if you're running alone on the school track and you suddenly feel like you're being watched, that could be your intuition telling you something. Your common sense would then tell you that it's a good idea to get back to where there are more people around.

## De-Escalating A Bad Situation

Attackers aren't always strangers who jump out of dark alleys. Sadly, teens can be attacked by people they know. That's where another important self-defense skill comes into play. This skill is something self-defense experts and negotiators call **de-escalation**.

About This Chapter: Text in this chapter is excerpted from "Self-Defense," © 1995–2016. The Nemours Foundation/KidsHealth®. Reprinted with permission.

De-escalating a situation means speaking or acting in a way that can prevent things from getting worse. The classic example of de-escalation is giving a robber your money rather than trying to fight or run. But de-escalation can work in other ways, too. For example, if someone harasses you when there's no one else around, you can de-escalate things by agreeing with him or her. You don't have to actually believe the taunts, of course, you're just using words to get you out of a tight spot. Then you can redirect the bully's focus ("Oops, I just heard the bell for third period"), and calmly walk away from the situation.

Something as simple as not losing your temper can de-escalate a situation. Learn how to manage your own anger effectively so that you can talk or walk away without using your fists or weapons.

Although de-escalation won't always work, it can only help matters if you remain calm and don't give the would-be attacker any extra ammunition. Whether it's a stranger or someone you thought you could trust, saying and doing things that don't threaten your attacker can give you some control.

# Reduce Your Risks

Another part of self-defense is doing things that can help you stay safe. Here are some tips from the National Crime Prevention Council (NCPC) and other experts:

- Understand your surroundings. Walk or hang out in areas that are open, well lit, and well traveled. Become familiar with the buildings, parking lots, parks, and other places you walk. Pay particular attention to places where someone could hide—such as stairways and bushes.

- Avoid shortcuts that take you through isolated areas.

- If you're going out at night, travel in a group.

- Make sure your friends and parents know your daily schedule (classes, sports practice, club meetings, etc.). If you go on a date or with friends for an after-game snack, let someone know where you're going and when you expect to return.

- Check out hangouts. Do they look safe? Are you comfortable being there? Ask yourself if the people around you seem to share your views on fun activities—if you think they're being reckless, move on.

- Be sure your body language shows a sense of confidence. Look like you know where you're going and act alert.

- When riding on public transportation, sit near the driver and stay awake. Attackers are looking for vulnerable targets.

- Carry a cell phone if possible. Make sure it's programmed with your parents' phone number.

- Be willing to report crimes in your neighborhood and school to the police.

# Take A Self-Defense Class

The best way—in fact the only way—to prepare yourself to fight off an attacker is to take a self-defense class. We'd love to give you all the right moves in an article, but some things you just have to learn in person.

A good self-defense class can teach you how to size up a situation and decide what you should do. Self-defense classes can also teach special techniques for breaking an attacker's grasp and other things you can do to get away. For example, attackers usually anticipate how their victim might react—that kick to the groin or jab to the eyes, for instance. A good self-defense class can teach you ways to surprise your attacker and catch him or her off guard.

One of the best things people take away from self-defense classes is self-confidence. The last thing you want to be thinking about during an attack is, "Can I really pull this self-defense tactic off?" It's much easier to take action in an emergency if you've already had a few dry runs.

A self-defense class should give you a chance to practice your moves. If you take a class with a friend, you can continue practicing on each other to keep the moves fresh in your mind long after the class is over.

Check out your local YMCA, community hospital, or community center for classes. If they don't have them, they may be able to tell you who does. Your PE teacher or school counselor may also be a great resource.

# Chapter 49
# Online Safety

How could we live without our smartphones, laptops, and other devices that allow us to go online? That's how most of us keep in touch with friends and family, take pictures, do our homework, do research, find out the latest news, and even shop.

But besides the millions of sites to visit and things to do, going online offers lots of ways to waste time—and even get into trouble. And just as in the non-cyber world, some people you encounter online might try to take advantage of you, steal your personal information, or harass or threaten you (called cyberbullying).

You've probably heard stories about people who got into trouble for something they did online—whether it was sending an inappropriate photograph by text message, joining in on some online bullying on a website or message app, or getting ripped off by someone they met through a website.

Because users can easily remain anonymous, some of the more popular websites and messaging apps might attract adults who pretend to be teens or kids. They'll sometimes ask visitors for pictures or information about themselves, their families, or where they live—information that shouldn't be given away.

Usually, the people who request personal information like home addresses, phone numbers, and email addresses use this information to fill mailboxes and answering machines with advertisements. In some cases, though, predators may use this information to begin illegal or indecent relationships or to harm a person or family.

About This Chapter: Text in this chapter is excerpted from "Online Safety," © 1995–2016. The Nemours Foundation/KidsHealth®. Reprinted with permission.

# Smart Surfing

First rule? Check your mood! Are you feeling upset or angry? Then this is not the time to be messaging or posting on a social media site. People don't always make good decisions or think straight when they're stressed out or upset. If you have to, call someone or go for a run instead before you start venting online.

Second rule: when you're on a website, try to remain as anonymous as possible. That means keeping all private information private. Here are some examples of private information that you should never allow the public to see:

- your full name

- any type of photograph (even of your pet!)

- your current location (some phones have automatic GPS apps built in that may need to be turned off)

- home or school address or the address of any of your family or friends

- phone numbers

- social security number

- passwords

- names of family members

- credit card numbers

Most trustworthy people and companies won't ask for this type of information online. So if others do, it's a red flag that they may be up to no good. Always check with a parent if you are unsure, especially when shopping online or signing up for a website or app.

Think carefully before you create an email address or screen name. Web experts recommend that you use a combination of letters and numbers in both—and that you don't identify whether you're male or female.

When using messaging or chat/video apps, use a nickname that's different from your screen name. That way, if you ever find yourself in a conversation that makes you uncomfortable, you can exit without having to worry that someone knows your screen name and can track you down via email. Some people who hang out with their friends online set up private chat rooms where only they and the people they invite can enter to chat.

Safety experts recommend that people keep online friendships in the virtual world. Meeting online friends face to face carries more risks than other types of friendships because it's so easy for people to pretend to be something they're not when you can't see them or talk in person. It's safer to Skype or video message with someone first, but even that can carry some risks. Check with a parent that this is a safe thing for you to be doing. They may want to meet some of your contacts or sit in on a conversation before they allow you to set up Skype by yourself.

If you ever get involved in any messaging or online chats that make you feel uncomfortable or in danger for any reason, exit and tell a parent or other adult right away so they can report the incident. You also can report it to the website of the National Center for Missing and Exploited Children—they have a form for reporting this type of incident called CyberTipline. They will then see that the info is forwarded to law enforcement officials for investigation.

# Cyberbullying

It's not just strangers who can make you feel uncomfortable. Cyberbullying refers to cruel or bullying messages sent to you online. These might be from former friends or other people you know. They can also be sent anonymously—in other words, on a website where everyone has a screen name, so teens being bullied might not even know who is bullying them.

If you get these bullying messages online, it's often better to ignore them rather than answer them. Cyberbullies, just like other bullies, might be looking for attention or a reaction. Plus, you never want to provoke bullies. By ignoring them, you can take away their power. You also can try to delete or block bullies so you no longer see their messages or texts.

Fortunately, most people never experience cyberbullying. But if you're getting cyberbullied and ignoring it doesn't make it stop, getting help from a parent, school counselor, or another trusted adult might be a good idea. That's especially true if the cyberbullying contains threats.

# Other Things To Consider

Although email is relatively private, hackers can still access it—or add you to their spam lists. Spam, like ads or harassing or offensive notes, is annoying. But spam blockers can keep your mailbox from getting clogged. Many service providers will help you block out or screen inappropriate emails if your parents agree to set up age-appropriate parental controls.

If you don't recognize the sender of a document or file that needs to be downloaded, delete it without opening it to avoid getting a virus on your device. Virus protection software is a must for every computer and should be updated regularly. You also can buy software that helps rid your computer of unwanted spyware programs that report what your computer is doing. Some service providers make software available to protect you from these and other online annoyances, such as blockers for those in-your-face pop-up ads.

When you're out and about with your devices, keep them secure. Don't let other people use your phone unless you're with them. Don't leave your phone where someone else might pick it up, and turn your laptop or tablet off when you're not using it. Don't make it easy for other people to get a look at your personal information.

Finally, remember that any pictures or text messages that you send could become "leaked," or public, as soon as you hit send. Think about whether the words you've written or the pictures you're about to share are ones that you would want other people reading or seeing. It's always better to be safe than sorry. A good rule is that if you wouldn't want your grandmother to see it or read it, you probably shouldn't send it or post it.

## Sexting: Don't Do It

You may have heard stories at school or in the news about people "sexting"—sending nude photos from mobile phones. Don't do it. Period. People who create, forward, or even save sexually explicit photos, videos, or messages are putting their friendships and reputations at risk. Worse yet, they could be breaking the law.

*Source: "Share With Care," Federal Trade Commission (FTC), August 2011.*

# Chapter 50
# Suicide Prevention

It's a sad truth that teens sometimes think about ending their lives. If you are feeling awful, you may think that suicide is the only answer—but it's not! Don't let suicide be the ending of your story. People want to help, and you can feel better.

---

### A Serious Issue
Suicide is one of the leading causes of teen deaths. Girls think about and attempt suicide more often than boys.

---

## What If I'm Thinking About Suicide?

**If you are thinking about suicide, get help right away.** You can contact the helpline by chat, or call **800-273-TALK (800-273-8255)**.

If there is an immediate risk, call 911 or go to the nearest hospital emergency department.

The people there can talk with you about your problems and help you make a plan to stay safe. They also can give you information about ways to get help in person.

**If you are in immediate danger of hurting yourself, call 911.** You also can go to the nearest hospital emergency department.

**Right now, your pain may feel too overwhelming to handle.** Suicide may feel like the only way to get relief when you're suffering. But people get past suicidal thoughts, and things

---

About This Chapter: This chapter includes text excerpted from "Feeling Suicidal," Girlshealth.gov, Office on Women's Health (OWH), January 7, 2015.

can get better. You can watch a video about a woman who survived suicide and went on to lead a wonderful life. Below, you can get some ideas on how to feel better.

**You can find ways to feel better.** Writing is one way to lower your pain. You might list things that you love or your hopes for the future. You also can hang up photos, messages, and other things that remind you that life is worth living. Also, reach out to people who care about you.

**Don't try using drugs or alcohol to feel better.** These things will not solve your problems. They will only create more problems.

# How Can I Help A Friend Who Has Suicidal Thoughts?

**If you think a friend is in immediate danger from suicide call 911 and do not leave him or her alone.**

If you think a friend is considering suicide but you're not sure, you can look for some signs. These include:

- Talking about not wanting to live
- Talking about looking for ways to die, like trying to get pills or a gun
- Talking about feeling hopeless or having no purpose
- Talking about feeling trapped or being in horrible pain
- Talking about being a burden to others
- Abusing drugs or alcohol
- Acting very nervous or on edge
- Doing dangerous things
- Sleeping a lot more than before or very little
- Not wanting to be around other people
- Changing quickly from one strong mood to another
- Doing some type of self-injury, like cutting
- Acting full of rage or talking about getting revenge

- Giving away favorite things

If a friend seems suicidal, ask the person to talk to you about what's going on. Listening shows you care. Remember, though, that you cannot help the person on your own. Encourage your friend to contact a suicide hotline. Suggest that your friend talk to an adult, and possibly offer to go with him or her.

Even if your friend does not want to talk with an adult, you need to tell one as quickly as possible. This can be a relative, school nurse, counselor, teacher, or coach, for example. If you are worried that your friend will be mad, remember that you are doing the right thing. You could save your friend's life.

# What If Someone I Know Attempts Or Dies By Suicide?

If someone you know attempts or dies by suicide, you may feel like it's your fault in some way. That's not true! You also may feel many different emotions, including anger, grief, or even emotional numbness. All of your feelings are okay. There is not a right or wrong way to feel.

If you are having trouble dealing with your feelings, talk to a trusted adult. You have suffered a terrible loss, but life can feel okay again. Reach out to people who care about you. Connecting is so important at this tough time.

# Why Do Some Teens Think About Suicide?

Some teens feel so terrible and overwhelmed that they think life will never get better. Some things that may cause these feelings include:

- The death of someone close
- Having depression or other mental health issues, such as an eating disorder, attention deficit hyperactivity disorder, or anxiety
- Having alcohol or drug problems
- Parents getting divorced
- Seeing a lot of anger and violence at home
- Having a hard time in school
- Being bullied

- Having problems with friends

- Experiencing a trauma like being raped or abused

- Being angry or heartbroken over a relationship break-up

- Feeling like you don't belong, either in your family or with friends

- Feeling rejected because of something about you, like being gay

- Having an ongoing illness or disability

- Feeling alone

- Feeling guilty or like a burden to other people

Also, teens sometimes may feel very bad for no one clear reason.

If you are suffering, know that things definitely can get better. You can learn ways to handle your feelings. You can work toward a much brighter future.

Turning to others can help you through tough times. If you don't feel a strong connection to relatives or friends, try talking to a school counselor, teacher, doctor, or another adult you trust.

Every teen feels anxiety, sadness, and confusion at some point. The important thing to remember is that life can get much better. There is always help out there for you or a friend.

# Chapter 51

# Your Legal Rights As A Victim Of Sexual Assault Or Domestic Abuse

## Violence Against Women

The U.S. Congress has passed two main laws related to violence against women, the Violence Against Women Act and the Family Violence Prevention and Services Act.

### The Violence Against Women Act

The Violence Against Women Act (VAWA) was the first major law to help government agencies and victim advocates work together to fight domestic violence, sexual assault, and other types of violence against women. It created new punishments for certain crimes and started programs to prevent violence and help victims. Over the years, the law has been expanded to provide more programs and services. Currently, some included items are:

- Violence prevention programs in communities

- Protections for victims who are evicted from their homes because of events related to domestic violence or stalking

- Funding for victim assistance services like rape crisis centers and hotlines

- Programs to meet the needs of immigrant women and women of different races or ethnicities

- Programs and services for victims with disabilities

---

About This Chapter: Text under with the heading "Violence Against Women" is excerpted from "Violence Against Women," Office on Women's Health (OWH), U.S. Department of Health and Human Services (HHS), September 30, 2015; Text beginning with the heading "Domestic Violence Laws" is excerpted from "Domestic Violence Laws," U.S. Department of Justice (DOJ), June 23, 2015.

- Legal aid for survivors of violence

- Services for children and teens

The National Advisory Committee on Violence Against Women works to help promote the goals and vision of VAWA. The committee is a joint effort between the U.S. Department of Justice (DOJ) and the U.S. Department of Health and Human Services (HHS). Examples of the committee's efforts include the Community Checklist initiative to make sure each community has domestic violence programs and the Toolkit to End Violence Against Women, which has chapters for specific audiences.

## The Family Violence Prevention And Services Act

The Family Violence Prevention and Services Act (FVPSA) provides the main federal funding to help victims of domestic violence and their dependents (such as children). Programs funded through FVPSA provide shelter and related help. They also offer violence prevention activities and try to improve how service agencies work together in communities. FVPSA works through a few main ways:

- **Formula Grants.** This money helps states, territories, and tribes create and support programs that work to help victims and prevent family violence. The amount of money is determined by a formula based partly on population. The states, territories, and tribes distribute the money to thousands of domestic violence shelters and programs.

- **The National Domestic Violence Hotline.** This is a 24-hour, confidential, toll-free hotline. Hotline staff connect the caller to a local service provider. Trained advocates provide support, information, referrals, safety planning, and crisis intervention in more than 170 languages to hundreds of thousands of domestic violence victims each year.

- **The Domestic Violence Prevention Enhancements and Leadership Through Alliances (DELTA) Program.** Like many public health problems, intimate partner violence is not simply an individual problem—it is a community problem. DELTA supports local programs that teach people ways to prevent violence.

# Domestic Violence Laws

Violence and abuse at the hands of a loved one is frightening, degrading and confusing. Have you experienced this violence and abuse? If so, you are a victim of domestic violence. You are also the victim of a crime. Despite your conflicting emotions, the legal system may be one of the most effective ways to protect yourself and your children.

In 1994, Congress passed the Violence Against Women Act ("VAWA"). This Act, and the 1996 additions to the Act, recognize that domestic violence is a national crime and that federal laws can help an overburdened state and local criminal justice system.

In 1994 and 1996, Congress also passed changes to the Gun Control Act making it a federal crime in certain situations for domestic abusers to possess guns. The majority of domestic violence cases will continue to be handled by your state and local authorities. In some cases, however, the federal laws and the benefits gained from applying these laws, may be the most appropriate course of action.

# Who Should I Call To Report A Possible Federal Crime?

For a possible Gun Control Act violation, please call your local Alcohol, Tobacco and Firearms ("ATF") Office. For a possible VAWA violation, please call your local Federal Bureau of Investigation ("FBI") Office. These violations are described in this chapter. If you are unsure of the violation, please call law enforcement or the Victim/Witness Coordinator.

# What Are The Federal Crimes And Penalties?

All the federal domestic violence crimes are felonies.

It is a federal crime under VAWA:

- to cross state lines or enter or leave Indian country and physically injure an "intimate partner" (18 U.S.C. Section 2261)

- to cross state lines to stalk or harass or to stalk or harass within the maritime or territorial lands of the United States (this includes military bases and Indian country) (18 U.S.C. Section 2261A)

- to cross state lines or enter or leave Indian country and violate a qualifying Protection Order (18 U.S.C. Section 2262)

It is a federal crime under the Gun Control Act:

- to possess a firearm and/or ammunition while subject to a qualifying Protection Order. 18 U.S.C. Section 922(g)(8)

- to possess a firearm and/or ammunition after conviction of a qualifying misdemeanor crime of domestic violence. 18 U.S.C. Section 922(g)(9)

A violation of the Gun Control Act, Sections 922(g)(8) and 922(g)(9), has a maximum prison term of ten years. A violation under VAWA, Sections 2261, 2261A and 2262, has a maximum prison term of five years to life, depending on the seriousness of the bodily injury caused by the defendant. In a VAWA case, the Court must order restitution to pay the victim the full amount of losses. These losses include costs for medical or psychological care, physical therapy, transportation, temporary housing, child care expenses, lost income, attorney's fees, costs incurred in obtaining a civil protection order, and any other losses suffered by the victim as a result of the offense. In a Gun Control Act case, the Court may order restitution.

Please keep a record of all expenses caused by the domestic violence crime.

## What Is A Qualifying Domestic Violence Misdemeanor?

Possession of a firearm and/or ammunition after conviction of a "qualifying" domestic violence misdemeanor is a federal crime under Section 922(g)(9). Generally, the misdemeanor will "qualify" if the conviction was for a crime committed by anintimate partner, parent or guardian of the victim that required the use or attempted use of physical force or the threatened use of a deadly weapon. In addition, Section 922(g)(9) imposes other legal requirements. The United States Attorney's Office (USAO) may examine your case and determine whether the prior domestic violence misdemeanor conviction qualifies under Section 922(g)(9).

## What Is A Qualifying Protection Order?

Possession of a firearm and/or ammunition while subject to a Protection Order, and interstate violation of a Protection Order are federal crimes if the Protection Order "qualifies" under Sections 2262 and 922(g)(8). Generally, a Protection Order will qualify under federal law if reasonable notice and an opportunity to be heard was given to the person against whom the Court's Order was entered and if the Order forbids future threats of violence. The United States Attorney's Office may evaluate your Order to see if it qualifies. Therefore you should keep copies of all Orders.

## Who Is An Intimate Partner?

Generally, the federal laws recognize an intimate partner as a spouse, a former spouse, a person who shares a child in common with the victim, or a person who cohabits or has cohabited with the victim.

# Can My Concerns Be Heard In Federal Court?

A victim in a VAWA case shall have the right to speak, if desired, to the Judge at a bail hearing to inform the Judge of any danger posed by the release of the defendant.

Any victim of a crime of violence shall also have the right to speak, if desired, at the time of sentencing, about the impact of the crime upon their life and that of their family.

# Crime Victims' Rights

A victim of a federal domestic violence crime has the following rights under 42 U.S.C. Section 10606(b):

- The right to be treated with fairness and with respect for the victim's dignity and privacy. The right to be reasonably protected from the accused offender. The right to be notified of court proceedings.

- The right to be present at all public Court proceedings related to the offense, unless the Court determines that testimony by the victim would be materially affected if the victim heard other testimony at trial.

- The right to confer with the attorney for the Government in the case.

- The right to restitution.

- The right to information about the conviction, sentencing, imprisonment and release of the offender.

In addition, victims of any domestic violence crime may be eligible for crime victim compensation which can include payment of medical expenses, lost wages, loss of support, and counseling for a victim and other family members. Other costs may also be considered. Contact a local victim services provider, or the U.S. Attorney's Victim/Witness Assistance Program for more information.

# Chapter 52
# Bullying And The Law

Although no federal law directly addresses bullying, in some cases, bullying overlaps with discriminatory harassment when it is based on race, national origin, color, sex, age, disability, or religion. When bullying and harassment overlap, federally-funded schools (including colleges and universities) have an obligation to resolve the harassment. When the situation is not adequately resolved, the U.S. Department of Education's (ED) Office for Civil Rights (OCR) and the U.S. Department of Justice's (DOJ) Civil Rights Division may be able to help.

## Are There Federal Laws That Apply To Bullying?

At present, no federal law directly addresses bullying. In some cases, bullying overlaps with discriminatory harassment which is covered under federal civil rights laws enforced by the U.S. Department of Education (ED) and the U.S. Department of Justice (DOJ). No matter what label is used (e.g., bullying, hazing, teasing), schools are obligated by these laws to address conduct that is:

- severe, pervasive or persistent

- creates a hostile environment at school. That is, it is sufficiently serious that it interferes with or limits a student's ability to participate in or benefit from the services, activities, or opportunities offered by a school

- based on a student's race, color, national origin, sex, disability, or religion

About This Chapter: This chapter includes text excerpted from "Federal Laws," Stopbullying.gov, U.S. Department of Health and Human Services (HHS), March 31, 2014.

# What Are The Federal Civil Rights Laws ED And DOJ Enforce?

- A school that fails to respond appropriately to harassment of students based on a protected class may be violating one or more civil rights laws enforced by the ED and the DOJ, including:

  - Title IV and Title VI of the Civil Rights Act of 1964

  - Title IX of the Education Amendments of 1972

  - Section 504 of the Rehabilitation Act of 1973

  - Titles II and III of the Americans with Disabilities Act

  - Individuals with Disabilities Education Act (IDEA)

# Do Federal Civil Rights Laws Cover Harassment Of LGBT Youth?

- Title IX and Title IV do not prohibit discrimination based solely on sexual orientation, but they protect all students, including students who are lesbian, gay, bisexual, and transgender (LGBT) or perceived to be LGBT, from sex-based harassment.

- Harassment based on sex and sexual orientation are not mutually exclusive. When students are harassed based on their actual or perceived sexual orientation, they may also be subjected to forms of sex discrimination recognized under Title IX.

# What Is An Example Of A Case Were Harassment Based On Sex And Sexual Orientation Overlap?

- A female high school student was spit on, slammed into lockers, mocked, and routinely called names because she did not conform to feminine stereotypes and because of her sexual orientation. The student had short hair, a deep voice, and wore male clothing. After the harassment started, she told some classmates she was a lesbian, and the harassment worsened. The school described the harassment as "sexual orientation harassment" in its incident reports and did not take any action.

- In this case, the student was harassed based on her non-conformity to gender stereotypes. In this case, then, although the school labeled the incident as "sexual orientation harassment," the harassment was also based on sex and covered under Title IX.

# What Are A School's Obligations Regarding Harassment Based On Protected Classes?

Anyone can report harassing conduct to a school. When a school receives a complaint they must take certain steps to investigate and resolve the situation.

- Immediate and appropriate action to investigate or otherwise determine what happened.

- Inquiry must be prompt, thorough, and impartial.

- Interview targeted students, offending students, and witnesses, and maintain written documentation of investigation

- Communicate with targeted students regarding steps taken to end harassment

- Check in with targeted students to ensure that harassment has ceased

- When an investigation reveals that harassment has occurred, a school should take steps reasonably calculated to:

  - end the harassment

  - eliminate any hostile environment

  - prevent harassment from recurring, and

  - prevent retaliation against the targeted student(s) or complainant(s)

# What Should A School Do To Resolve A Harassment Complaint?

- Appropriate responses will depend on the facts of each case.

- School must be an active participant in responding to harassment and should take reasonable steps when crafting remedies to minimize burdens on the targeted students.

- Possible responses include:

  - Develop, revise, and publicize:

    - policy prohibiting harassment and discrimination

    - grievance procedures for students to file harassment complaints

    - contact information for Title IX/Section 504/Title VI coordinators

- Implement training for staff and administration on identifying and addressing harassment.

- Provide monitors or additional adult supervision in areas where harassment occurs.

- Determine consequences and services for harassers, including whether discipline is appropriate.

- Limit interactions between harassers and targets.

- Provide harassed student an additional opportunity to obtain a benefit that was denied (e.g., retaking a test/class).

- Provide services to a student who was denied a benefit (e.g., academic support services).

## Are There Resources For Schools To Assist With Resolving Harassment Complaints?

The DOJ's Community Relations Service is the Department's "peacemaker" for community conflicts and tensions arising from differences of race, color and national origin and to prevent and respond to violent hate crimes committed on the basis of: gender, gender identity, sexual orientation, religion, disability, race, color, and national origin. It is a free, impartial, confidential and voluntary Federal Agency that offers mediation, conciliation, technical assistance, and training.

# Part Five
If You Need More Information

# Chapter 53

# Abuse And Violence: A Statistical Summary

## Child Abuse And Neglect: Consequences

Child abuse and neglect affect children's health now and later, and costs to our country are significant. Neglect, physical abuse, custodial interference, and sexual abuse are types of child maltreatment that can lead to poor physical and mental health well into adulthood.

### Prevalence

- An estimated 702,000 children were confirmed by child protective services as being victims of abuse and neglect in 2014.

- At least one in four children have experienced child neglect or abuse (including physical, emotional, and sexual) at some point in their lives, and one in seven children experienced abuse or neglect in 2014.

### Physical

In 2014, approximately 1,580 children died from abuse and neglect across the country—a rate of 2.13 deaths per 100,000 children.

---

About This Chapter: Text under the heading "Child Abuse And Neglect: Consequences" is excerpted from "Violence Prevention: Child Abuse And Neglect: Consequences," Centers for Disease Control and Prevention (CDC), March 28, 2016; Text under the heading "School Violence" is excerpted from "Understanding School Violence: Factsheet," Centers for Disease Control and Prevention (CDC), 2016; Text under the heading "Bullying" is excerpted from "Understanding Bullying: Factsheet," Centers for Disease Control and Prevention (CDC), 2016; Text under the heading "Youth Violence" is excerpted from "Understanding Youth Violence: Factsheet," Centers for Disease Control and Prevention (CDC), 2015; Text under the heading "Teen Dating Violence" is excerpted from "Understanding Teen Dating Violence: Factsheet," Centers for Disease Control and Prevention (CDC), 2016.

## Psychological

In one long-term study, as many as 80 percent of young adults who had been abused met the diagnostic criteria for at least one psychiatric disorder at age 21. These young adults exhibited many problems, including depression, anxiety, eating disorders, and suicide attempts.

## Behavioral

- Those with a history of child abuse and neglect are 1.5 times more likely to use illicit drugs, especially marijuana, in middle adulthood.

- Studies have found abused and neglected children to be at least 25 percent more likely to experience problems such as delinquency, teen pregnancy, and low academic achievement. Similarly, a longitudinal study found that physically abused children were at greater risk of being arrested as juveniles, being a teen parent, and less likely to graduate high school.

- A National Institute of Justice (NIJ) study indicated that being abused or neglected as a child increased the likelihood of arrest as a juvenile by 59%. Abuse and neglect also increased the likelihood of adult criminal behavior by 28 percent and violent crime by 30%.

# School Violence

School violence is youth violence that occurs on school property, on the way to or from school or school-sponsored events, or during a schools-sponsored event. A young person can be a victim, a perpetrator, or a witness of school violence. School violence may also involve or impact adults.

Youth violence includes various behaviors. Some violent acts—such as bullying, pushing, and shoving—can cause more emotional harm than physical harm. Other forms of violence, such as gang violence and assault (with or without weapons), can lead to serious injury or even death.

School associated violent deaths are rare.

- 31 homicides of school-age youth, ages 5 to 18 years, occurred at school during the 2012–2013 school year.

- Of all youth homicides, less than 2.6 percent occur at school, and this percentage has been relatively stable for the past decade.

In 2014, there were about 486,400 nonfatal violent victimizations at school among students 12 to 18 years of age.

Approximately 9 percent of teachers report that they have been threatened with injury by a student from their school; 5 percent of school teachers reported that they had been physically attacked by a student from their school.

In 2013, 12 percent of students ages 12–18 reported that gangs were present at their school during the school year.

In a 2015 nationally representative sample of youth in grades 9–12:

- 7.8 percent reported being in a physical fight on school property in the 12 months before the survey.

- 5.6 percent reported that they did not go to school on one or more days in the 30 days before the survey because they felt unsafe at school or on their way to or from school.

- 4.1 percent reported carrying a weapon (gun, knife or club) on school property on one or more days in the 30 days before the survey.

- 6.0 percent reported being threatened or injured with a weapon on school property one or more times in the 12 months before the survey.

- 20.2 percent reported being bullied on school property and 15.5 percent reported being bullied electronically during the 12 months before the survey.

# Bullying

Bullying is a form of youth violence. Centers for Disease Control and Prevention (CDC) defines bullying as any unwanted aggressive behavior(s) by another youth or group of youths who are not siblings or current dating partners that involves an observed or perceived power imbalance and is repeated multiple times or is highly likely to be repeated. Bullying may inflict harm or distress on the targeted youth including physical, psychological, social, or educational harm.

Bullying can include aggression that is physical (hitting, tripping), verbal (name calling, teasing), or relational/ social (spreading rumors, leaving out of group). A young person can be a perpetrator, a victim, or both (also known as "bully/victim").

Bullying can also occur through technology and is called electronic aggression or cyber-bullying. Electronic aggression is bullying that occurs through e-mail, a chat room, instant messaging, a website, text messaging, or videos or pictures posted on websites or sent through cell phones

Bullying is widespread in the United States.

- In a 2015 nationwide survey, 20 percent of high school students reported being bullied on school property in the 12 months preceding the survey.

- An estimated 16 percent of high school students reported in 2015 that they were bullied electronically in the 12 months before the survey.

# Youth Violence

Youth violence refers to harmful behaviors that can start early and continue into young adulthood. The young person can be a victim, an offender, or a witness to the violence.

Youth violence includes various behaviors. Some violent acts—such as bullying, slapping, or hitting—can cause more emotional harm than physical harm. Others, such as robbery and assault (with or without weapons), can lead to serious injury or even death.

Youth violence is widespread in the United States. It is the third leading cause of death for young people between the ages of 15 and 24.

- In 2012, 4,787 young people aged 10 to 24 years were victims of homicide—an average of 13 each day.

- Over 599,000 young people aged 10 to 24 years had physical assault injuries treated in U.S. emergency departments—an average of 1642 each day.

- In a 2013 nationwide survey, about 24.7 percent of high school students reported being in a physical fight in the 12 months before the survey.

- About 17.9 percent of high school students in 2013 reported taking a weapon to school in the 30 days before the survey.

- In 2013, 19.6 percent of high school students reported being bullied on school property and 14.8 percent reported being bullied electronically.

- Each year, youth homicides and assault-related injuries result in an estimated $16 billion in combined medical and work loss costs.

# Teen Dating Violence

Dating violence is a type of intimate partner violence. It occurs between two people in a close relationship. The nature of dating violence can be physical, emotional, or sexual.

- Dating violence is a widespread issue that has serious long-term and short-term effects. Many teens do not report it because they are afraid to tell friends and family.

- Among high school students who dated, 21 percent of females and 10 percent of males experienced physical and/ or sexual dating violence.

- Among adult victims of rape, physical violence, and/ or stalking by an intimate partner, 22 percent of women and 15 percent of men first experienced some form of partner violence between 11 and 17 years of age.

# Chapter 54
# Directory Of Abuse And Violence Resources

## Teen Dating Violence Resource List

### Hotlines

### *National Domestic Violence Hotline*
P.O. Box 161810
Austin, TX 78716
Toll-Free: 800-799-SAFE (800-799-7233)
Phone: 512-453-8117
Toll-Free TTY: 800-787-3224
Website: www.thehotline.org

### *National Hopeline Network*
Toll-Free: 800-SUICIDE (800-784-2433)
Website: hopeline.com
E-mail: info@iamalive.org

### *National Runaway Hotline*
3141B N. Lincoln
Chicago, IL 60657
Toll-Free: 800-RUNAWAY (800-786-2929)
Phone: 773-880-9860
Fax: 773-929-5150
Website: 1800runaway.org

---

Resources in this chapter were compiled from several sources deemed reliable, November 2016.

### Rape Abuse and Incest National Network (RAINN)

Toll-Free: 800-656-HOPE (800-656-4673)
Website: www.rainn.org

## Domestic Violence Organizations

### Family Violence Prevention Fund (FVPF)

383 Rhode Island St.
Ste. 304
San Francisco, CA 94103-5133
Phone: 415-252-8900
Fax: 415-252-8991
Website: www.endabuse.org
E-mail: info@endabuse.org

### National Coalition Against Domestic Violence (NCADV)

One Bdwy.,
Ste. B210
Denver, CO 80203
Phone: 303-839-1852
Fax: 303-831-9251
Website: www.ncadv.org
E-mail: mainoffice@ncadv.org

### National Resource Center on Domestic Violence (NRCDV)

6041 Linglestown Rd.
Harrisburg, PA 17112
Toll-Free: 800-537-2238
TTY: 800-787-3224
Website: www.nrcdv.org
E-mail: nrcdvTA@nrcdv.org

### Pennsylvania Coalition Against Domestic Violence and National Resource Center (PCADV)

3605 Vartan Way
Ste. 101
Harrisburg, PA 17110
Toll-Free: 800-932-4632
Phone: 717-545-6400
Toll-Free TTY: 800-553-2508
Website: www.pcadv.org

## Teen Dating Violence

### Break the Cycle

P.O. Box 811334
Los Angeles, CA 90081
Toll-Free: 888-988-TEEN (888-988-8336)
Phone: 424-265-7346
Website: www.breakthecycle.org
E-mail: info@breakthecycle.org

### Girls Inc.

120 Wall St.
New York, NY 10005-3902
Phone: 212-509-2000
Website: www.girlsinc.org
E-mail: communications@girlsinc.org

### Peace Over Violence

Metro Headquarters
1015 Wilshire Blvd.
Ste. 200
Los Angeles, CA 90017
Phone: 213-955-9090
TTY: 213-955-9095
Fax: 213-955-9093
Website: www.peaceoverviolence.org
E-mail: info@peaceoverviolence.org

## Lesbian, Gay, Bisexual, Transgendered, Queer (LGBTQ) Youth

### Community United Against Violence (CUAV)

427 S. Van Ness Ave.
San Francisco, CA 94103
Phone: 415-777-5500
Fax: 415-777-5565
Website: www.cuav.org
E-mail: info@cuav.org

### Parents, Families, and Friends of Lesbians and Gays (PFLAG)

1726 M St, N.W.
Ste. 400
Washington, DC 20036
Phone: 202-467-8180
Fax: 202-467-8194
Website: www.pflag.org
E-mail: info@pflag.org

## Teen Pregnancy

### American College of Obstetricians and Gynecologists (ACOG)

P.O. Box 70620
Washington, DC 20024-9998
Phone: 202-863-2487
Fax: 202-484-3917
Website: www.acog.org
E-mail: adolhlth@acog.org

## Sexual Assault

### FaithTrust Institute

2414 S.W. Andover St.
Ste. D208
Seattle, WA 98106
Phone: 206-634-1903
Fax: 206-634-0115
Website: www.faithtrustinstitute.org
E-mail: cpsdv@cpsdv.org

### Rape Abuse and Incest National Network (RAINN)

635 B Pennsylvania Ave. S.E.
Washington, DC 20003
Toll-Free: 800-656-HOPE (800-656-4673)
Fax: 202-544-3556
Website: www.rainn.org
Online Chat: online.rainn.org

## Office on Violence Against Women (OVW)

U.S. Department of Justice (DOJ)
950 Pennsylvania Ave. N.W.
Washington, DC 20530-0001
Phone: 202-353-1555
Website: www.justice.gov/ovw

## Additional Abuse And Violence Resources

## American Bar Association

Chicago Headquarters
321 N. Clark St.
Chicago, IL 60654
Toll-Free: 800-285-2221
Phone: 312-988-5000
Website: www.abanet.org

## American Humane

1400 16th St. N.W., Ste. 360
Washington, DC 20036
Toll-Free: 800-227-4645
Website: www.americanhumane.org
E-mail: info@americanhumane.org

## Child Welfare Information Gateway

Children's Bureau/ACYF
330 C St. S.W.
Washington, DC 20201
Toll-Free: 800-394-3366
Fax: 703-385-3206
Website: www.childwelfare.gov
E-mail: info@childwelfare.gov

## Internet Crimes Against Children (ICAC) Task Force Program

Office of Juvenile Justice and Delinquency Prevention (OJJDP), U.S. Department of Justice
(DOJ)
810 Seventh St. N.W.
Washington, DC 20531
Phone: 202-307-5933
Website: www.ojjdp.ncjrs.gov/programs/ProgSummary.asp?pi=3

### The Kempe Foundation

The Gary Pavilion at Children's Hospital Colorado
13123 E., 16th Ave. Anschutz Medical Campus,
Ste. B390
Aurora, CO 80045
Phone: 303-864-5300
Website: www.kempe.org

### National Center for Missing and Exploited Children

699 Prince St.
Charles B. Wang International Children's Bldg.
Alexandria, VA 22314
Toll-Free: 800-THE-LOST (800-843-5678)
Phone: 703-224-2150
Fax: 703-224-2122
Website: www.missingkids.com

### National Center for Victims of Crime

2000 M St. N.W., Ste. 480
Washington, DC 20036
Phone: 202-467-8700
Fax: 202-467-8701
Website: victimsofcrime.org

### Office for Victims of Crime

U.S. Department of Justice (DOJ)
810 Seventh St. N.W.
Washington, DC 20531
Toll-Free TTY: 800-877-8339
Website: www.ovc.gov

### Prevent Child Abuse America

228 S. Wabash Ave.
10th Fl.
Chicago, IL 60604
Toll-Free: 800-CHILDREN (800-244-5373)
Phone: 312-663-3520
Fax: 312-939-8962
Website: www.preventchildabuse.org
E-mail: mailbox@preventchildabuse.org

## *Start Strong*

Futures Without Violence
100 Montgomery St.
San Francisco, CA 94129
Phone: 415-678-5500
Website: startstrong.futureswithoutviolence.org
E-mail: info@startstrongteens.org

# Chapter 55

# Victims Of Abuse And Violence: Where To Go For Help

## Child Abuse

### *Childhelp*

4350 E. Camelback Rd.
Bldg. F250
Phoenix, AZ 85018
Toll-Free: 800-422-4453
Phone: 480-922-8212
Website: www.childhelp.org

### *Childsafe*

320 Cathedral St.
Baltimore, MD 21201
Toll-Free: 800-4-A-CHILD (800-422-4453)
Phone: 410-547-5348
Website: www.childsafeeducation.com
E-mail: assistance@archbalt.org

### *Prevent Child Abuse America*

228 S. Wabash Ave., 10th Fl.
Chicago, IL 60604
Phone: 312-663-3520
Fax: 312-939-8962
Website: www.preventchildabuse.org
E-mail: mailbox@preventchildabuse.org

Resources in this chapter were compiled from several sources deemed reliable, November 2016.

# Child Sexual Abuse

### Stop It Now!
351 Pleasant St.
Ste. B-319
Northampton, MA 01060
Toll-Free: 888-PREVENT (888-773-8368)
Phone: 413-587-3500
Website: www.stopitnow.org

### Washington Coalition of Sexual Assault Programs (WCSAP)
4317 6th Ave. S.E.
Ste. 102
Olympia, WA 98503
Phone: 360-754-7583
TTY: 360-709-0305
Fax: 360-786-8707
Website: www.wcsap.org
E-mail: info@wcsap.org

# Family Violence

### National Domestic Violence Hotline
P.O. Box 161810
Austin, TX 78716
Toll-Free: 800-799-7233
Phone: 512-453-8117
TTY: 800-787-3224
Website: www.thehotline.org
E-mail: development@ndvh.org

# Missing/Abducted Children

### Child Find Of America
P.O. Box 277
New Paltz, NY 12561
Toll-Free: 800-I-AM-LOST (800-426-5678)
Phone: 845-883-6060
Website: childfindofamerica.org
E-mail: information@childfindofamerica.org

### National Center For Missing And Exploited Children
699 Prince St.
Alexandria, VA 22314-3175
Toll-Free: 800-THE-LOST (800-843-5678)
Phone: 703-224-2150
Fax: 703-224-2122
Website: www.missingkids.com

### Operation Lookout National Center For Missing Youth
6320 Evergreen Way, Ste. 201
Everett, WA 98203
Phone: 425-771-7335
Website: www.operationlookout.org

# Rape/Incest

### Rape And Incest National Network
Toll-Free: 800-656-4673
Website: www.rainn.org

# Youth In Trouble / Runaways

### National Runaway Safeline
3141B N. Lincoln
Chicago, IL 60657
Toll-Free: 800-RUNAWAY (800-786-2929)
Phone: 773-880-9860
Fax: 773-929-5150
Website: www.1800runaway.org

# Crime Victims

### National Center For Victims Of Crime
2000 M St. N.W.
Ste. 480
Washington, DC 20036
Phone: 202-467-8700
Fax: 202-467-8701
Website: victimsofcrime.org

# Chapter 56

# How And Where To Report Child Abuse

## Alabama

### *Department of Human Resources*
50 N. Ripley St.
Gordon Persons Bldg, Ste. 2104
Montgomery, AL 36130
Phone: 334-242-1310
Fax: 334-353-1115
Website: dhr.alabama.gov

## Alaska

### *Department of Health and Social Services*
office of The Commissioner
3601 C St., Ste. 902
Anchorage, AK 99503-5923
Phone: 907-269-7800
Fax: 907-269-0060
Website: dhss.alaska.gov
E-mail: Scheduling.dhss@alaska.gov

---

Resources in this chapter were compiled from several sources deemed reliable, November 2016.

# Arizona

### Department of Child Safety (DCS)
P.O. Box 6030
Phoenix, AZ 85005-6030
Phone: 602-255-2500
Website: dcs.az.gov
E-mail: DCSGeneralInquiries@azdes.gov

# Arkansas

### Department of Human Services
Donaghey Pl.
P.O. Box 1437
Little Rock, AR 72203
Phone: 501-682-1001
TDD: 501-682-8820
TTY: 800-285-1131
Website: humanservices.arkansas.gov

# California

### Department of Social Services (CDSS)
744 P St.
MS 9-9-61
Sacramento, CA 95814
Phone: 916-651-8848
Website: www.cdss.ca.gov
E-mail: iso@dss.ca.gov

# Colorado

### Department of Human Services
1575 Sherman St., 2nd fl.
Denver, CO 80203
Toll-Free: 844-CO-4-KIDS (844-264-5437)
Phone: 303-866-5932
Fax: 303-866-5563
Website: www.state.co.us

# Connecticut

### Department of Children and Families

505 Hudson St.
Hartford, CT 06106
Toll-Free: 866-637-4737
Phone: 860-550-6301
Website: www.ct.gov
E-mail: Commissioner.dcf@ct.gov

# Delaware

### Department of Services For Children

1825 Faulkland Rd.
Wilmington, DE 19805-1195
Toll-Free: 800-292-9582
Website: kids.delaware.gov
E-mail: info.dscyf@state.de.us

# District of Columbia

### Child and Family Services Agency (CFSA)

200 I St. S.E.
Washington, DC 20003
Phone: 202-442-6100
Fax: 202-727-6505
Website: cfsa.dc.gov
E-mail: cfsa@dc.gov

# Florida

### Department of Children & Families

Headquarters
1317 Winewood Blvd.
Bldg. 1, Rm. 202
Tallahassee, FL 32399-0700
Toll-Free: 800-962-2873
Phone: 850-487-1111
Toll-Free TTY: 800-453-5145
Toll-Free Fax: 800-914-0004
Website: reportabuse.dcf.state.fl.us/

# Georgia

### Division of Family and Children Services (DFCS)

Toll-Free: 855-GA CHILD (855-422-4453)
Phone: 404-657-3550
Website: dfcs.dhs.georgia.gov
E-mail: CPSISSelfCheck@dhs.ga.gov

# Hawaii

### Department of Human Services Social Services

1390 Miller St., Rm. 209
Honolulu, HI 96813
Toll-Free: 800-494-3991
Phone: 808-586-4993
Fax: 808-586-4890
Website: humanservices.hawaii.gov
E-mail: dhs@dhs.hawaii.gov

# Idaho

### Department of Health and Welfare

1720 N. Westgate Dr
Boise, ID 83704
Toll-Free: 855-552-KIDS (855-552-5437)
Website: healthandwelfare.idaho.gov

# Illinois

### Department of Children and Family Services

406 E. Monroe St.
Springfield, IL 62701
Toll-Free: 800-25-ABUSE (252-2873)
Toll-Free TTY: 800-358-5117
Website: www.illinois.gov

# Indiana

### *Indiana Child Support Bureau*
Inquiry Unit MS 11
402 W. Washington St.
Indianapolis, IN 46204
Toll-Free: 800-800-5556
Phone: 317-233-5437
Website: www.in.gov/dcs/support.htm
E-mail: childsupportwebinquires.dcs@dcs.in.gov

# Iowa

### *Department of Human Services*
Toll-Free: 800-362-2178
Website: dhs.iowa.gov/child-abuse

# Kansas

### *Department for Children and Families*
555 S. Kansas Ave.
Topeka, KS 66603
Toll-Free: 888-369-4777
Phone: 785-296-3271
TTY: 785-296-1491
Website: www.dcf.ks.gov

# Kentucky

### *Cabinet for Health and Family Services (CHFS)*
275 E. Main St.
Frankfort, KY 40621
Toll-Free: 877-KYSAFE1 (877-597-2331)
Phone: 502-564-5497
Fax: 502-564-9523
Website: chfs.ky.gov
E-mail: Sherry.Carnahan@ky.gov

# Louisiana

### Department of Children & Family Services (DCFS)
627 N. Fourth St.
Baton Rouge, LA 70802
Toll-Free: 855-4LA-KIDS (855-452-5437)
Website: dss.louisiana.gov

# Maine

### Office of Child and Family Services (OCFS)
2 Anthony Ave.
Augusta, ME 04333-011
Toll-Free: 888-568-1112
Phone: 207- 624-7900
Fax: 207-287-5282
Website: www.maine.gov

# Maryland

### Maryland Department of Human Resources
Child Protective Services
311 W. Saratoga St.
Baltimore, MD 21201
Toll-Free: 800-332-6347
Toll-Free TTY: 800-925-4434
Website: dhr.maryland.gov/child-protective-services

# Massachusetts

### Executive Office of Health and Human Services (EOHHS)
1 Ashburton Pl.
11th Fl.
Boston, MA 02108
Toll-Free: 800-792-5200
Phone: 617-573-1600
Website: www.mass.gov

# Michigan

### Michigan Department of Health & Human Services (MDHHS)
333 S. Grand Ave.
P.O. Box 30195
Lansing, MI 48909
Toll-Free: 855-444-3911
Phone: 517-373-3740
Fax: 616-977-1154
Website: www.michigan.gov

# Minnesota

### Department of Human Services (DHS)
Children and Family Services
P.O. Box 64943
St. Paul, MN 55164-0943
Phone: 651-431-2000
Toll-Free TTY: 800-627-3529
Website: www.mn.gov/dhs

# Mississippi

### Mississippi Department of Human Services
750 N. State St.
Jackson, MS 39202
Toll-Free: 800-345-6347
Website: www.mdhs.state.ms.us

# Missouri

### Department of Social Services (DSS)
Division of Youth Services (DYS)
3418 Knipp, Ste. A-1
P.O. Box 447
Jefferson City, MO 65102-0447
Toll-Free: 800-392-3738
Phone: 573-751-3324
Fax: 573-526-4494
Website: dss.mo.gov
E-mail: AskDYS@dss.mo.gov

# Nebraska

### Department of Health & Human Services
301 Centennial Mall S.
Lincoln, NE 68509
Phone: 402-471-3121
Website: dhhs.ne.gov
E-mail: DHHS.Webmaster@Nebraska.gov

# Nevada

### Division of Child & Family Services
4126 Technology Way
3rd Fl.
Carson City, NV 89706
Toll-Free: 800-992-5757
Phone: 775-684-4400
Fax: 775-684-4455
Website: dcfs.nv.gov
E-mail: systems.advocate@dcfs.nv.gov

# New Hampshire

### Department of Health and Human Services
129 Pleasant St.
Concord, NH 03301-3852
Toll-Free: 800-894-5533
Website: www.dhhs.nh.gov

# New Jersey

### Department of Children and Families
50 E. State St.
2nd fl. P.O. Box 729
Trenton, NJ 08625-0729
Toll-Free: 855-INFO-DCF (855-463-6323)
Website: www.nj.gov
E-mail: askdcf@dcf.state.nj.us

# New Mexico

### Children Youth & Families Department (CYFD)
Toll-Free: 855-333-SAFE (855-333-7233)
Phone: 505-827-8400
Website: cyfd.org

# New York

### Office of Children and Family Services (OCFS)
52 Washington St.
Rensselaer, NY 12144-2834
Toll-Free: 800-342-3720
Phone: 518-473-7793
TDD: 800-369-2437
Fax: 518-486-7550
Website: ocfs.ny.gov

# North Carolina

### DHHS- Division of Social Services
820 S. Boylan Ave.
Dorothea Dix Campus, McBryde Bldg.
Raleigh, NC 27603
Phone: 919-527-6335
Fax: 919-334-1018
Website: www.ncdhhs.gov

# North Dakota

### Department of Human Services
600 E. Blvd. Ave.
Bismarck, ND 58505-0250
Website: www.nd.gov

# Ohio

## *Central Registry on Child Abuse and Neglect*
Department Of Job And Family Services
Office of Families and Children
P.O. Box 183204
Columbus, OH 43218-3204
Toll-Free: 855 O-H-CHILD (855 642-4453)
Phone: 614-752-1298
Website: jfs.ohio.gov/ocf/reportchildabuseandneglect.stm
E-mail: barbara.parker@jfs.ohio.gov; janice.blue@jfs.ohio.gov

# Oklahoma

## *The Office of Child Abuse Prevention*
Oklahoma State Department of Health (OSDH)
1000 N.E. 10th St.
Oklahoma City, OK 73117-1299
Toll-Free: 800-522-3511
Phone: 405-271-7611
Fax: 405-271-1011
Website: www.ok.gov

# Oregon

## *Department of Human Services*
500 Summer St. N.E.
Salem, OR 97301
Toll-Free: 855-503-SAFE (7233)
Website: www.oregon.gov

# Pennsylvania

## *Child Welfare Services*
Department of Human Services
P.O. Box 2675
Harrisburg, PA 17105-2675
Toll-Free: 800-932-0313
TDD: 866-872-1677
Website: www.dhs.pa.gov/citizens/childwelfareservices/index.htm

# Rhode Island

### Department of Children, Youth and Families (DYCF)
101 Friendship St.
Providence, RI 02903-3716
Phone: 401-528-3502
Website: www.dcyf.ri.gov

# South Carolina

### Department of Social Services
1535 Confederate Ave.
Columbia, SC 29201-1915
Website: dss.sc.gov

# South Dakota

### Department of Social Services
700 Governors Dr.
Pierre, SD 57501
Toll-Free: 800-694-8518
Phone: 605-773-3165
Website: dss.sd.gov

# U.S. Virgin Islands

### Department of Human Services
1303 Hospital Ground Knud Hansen Complex
Bldg. A
St. Thomas, VI 00802
Phone: 340-774-0930
Website: www.dhs.gov

# Utah

### Child and Family Services
195 N. 1950 W.
Salt Lake City, UT 84116
Toll-Free: 855-323-323
Phone: 801-538-4100
Fax: 801-538-3993
Website: dcfs.utah.gov
E-mail: CAROLMILLER@utah.gov

# Vermont

### *Department for Children and Families*
280 State Dr.
HC 1 N.
Waterbury, VT 05671-1080
Phone: 802-241-0927
Website: dcf.vermont.gov

# Virginia

### *Department of Social Services*
801 E. Main St.
Richmond, VA 23219
Toll-Free: 800-552-3431
Phone: 804-726-7000
Website: www.dss.virginia.gov

# Washington

### *State Department of Social And Health Services*
P.O. Box 45131
Olympia, WA 98504-45131
Toll-Free: 866-363-4276
TTY: 800-624-6186
Fax: 888-338-7410
Website: www.dshs.wa.gov

# West Virginia

### *Bureau For Children and Families*
350 Capitol St., Rm. 730
Charleston, WV 25301
Toll-Free: 800-352-6513
Phone: 304-558-0628
Fax: 304-558-4194
Website: www.dhhr.wv.gov

# Wisconsin

## *Department of Children and Families*

201 E. Washington Ave.
2nd fl. P.O. Box 8916
Madison, WI 53708-8916
Phone: 608-267-3905
Fax: 608-266-6836
Website: dcf.wisconsin.gov
E-mail: dcfweb@wisconsin.gov

# Index

# Index

Page numbers that appear in *Italics* refer to tables or illustrations. Page numbers that have a small 'n' after the page number refer to citation information shown as Notes. Page numbers that appear in **Bold** refer to information contained in boxes within the chapters.

# O